Praise for *Outsmarting Obesity*

"This well-researched book is rich with content yet remarkably accessible. It does indeed 'serve as an introductory course on the science of obesity.' It reviews numerous contributors to weight gain, from epigenetics to seemingly mundane behaviors. From these insights, practical and uncomplicated strategies for weight management emerge. This book can greatly serve both the individual struggling with obesity and the clinician faced with the challenge of the obesity epidemic."

—Jeremy E. Korman, MD, FACS, medical director, Marina Weight Management Center of Cedars-Sinai

"There are a lot of excellent books on the market about obesity, but this one offers the simplest and most relatable solution to our exploding obesity epidemic. It is well researched, well written, scientifically sound, and follows the science of nutrition and the truth about weight loss. The book is easy to read whether you're a health professional or a layperson. It covers the myths of weight gain/loss and gives practical advice. This is the best book of its kind on the market, and the only one you need to read if you want to understand how you can lose weight, conquer obesity without drugs, and improve your overall health. Dr. Lonky approaches everything from a medical model, showing why modern medicine has gotten obesity so wrong and how we can finally get it right."

—Lyssa Weiss, MS, RD, CDN, author of *The Skinny Jeans Diet* and owner of Skinny Jeans Nutrition, LLC

"Dr. Stewart Lonky's *Outsmarting Obesity* is a brilliant, science-driven revelation that delves deep into the complexities of obesity. With masterful prose, Lonky navigates through the heart of today's most pressing epidemic, offering timely insights and innovative strategies. *Outsmarting Obesity* is not just a book; it's a roadmap for a healthier future. A must-read for anyone concerned about their health and well-being."

—John M. Kennedy, MD, FACC, author of
The Heart Health Bible and *The 15 Minute Heart Cure*

"'Everything you always wanted to know about obesity' pretty much describes Dr. Stewart Lonky's highly readable new book, *Outsmarting Obesity*. Lonky identifies the matrix of factors contributing to obesity as the essential precursor to outsmarting it. He also provides a four-step program to combat the epidemic, mainly focusing on toxic compounds and chemicals in your household and toxic eating behaviors. This is essential reading for anybody who has a weight problem or cares about someone who does."

—Bill Tarrant, former foreign correspondent for *Reuters*

"*Outsmarting Obesity* is an exceptionally easy read—not preachy, and in language the average person can easily understand. Sit down and read it or take it an easy chapter at a time. Dr. Lonky offers options that will help put you in the weight loss column."

—Bob Nesoff, author, travel columnist, talk radio host, and cofounder and former national president of the North American Travel Journalists Association

"Author Stewart Lonky has crafted an enlightening and empowering work that combines plenty of valid scientific research with practical, actionable advice for the everyday person. The clear, crisp narrative style is free of jargon and always aims to be accessible, and it illuminates the complexities of obesity while demystifying a lot of common misconceptions. Harnessing cutting-edge science alongside common-sense strategies, Lonky and his fellow contributor Chris Talley offer a roadmap for sustainable weight management that is realistic and achievable. . . . Overall, *Outsmarting Obesity* is a highly recommended read for people seeking realistic weight loss and lifestyle coaching."

—*Readers' Favorite*

STEWART LONKY, MD

With Contributions by **CHRIS TALLEY, MS**

Foreword by **STEPHEN SINATRA, MD**

OUTSMARTING
OBESITY

A Doctor Reveals Why We Gain Weight,
Why It Matters, and What We Can Do About It

GREENLEAF
BOOK GROUP PRESS

This book is intended as a reference volume only, not as a medical manual. The information given here is designed to help you make informed decisions about your health. It is not intended as a substitute for any treatment that may have been prescribed by your doctor. If you suspect that you have a medical problem, you should seek competent medical help. You should not begin a new health regimen without first consulting a medical professional.

Published by Greenleaf Book Group Press
Austin, Texas
www.gbgpress.com

Distributed by Greenleaf Book Group

For ordering information or special discounts for bulk purchases, please contact Greenleaf Book Group at PO Box 91869, Austin, TX 78709, 512.891.6100.

Design and composition by Greenleaf Book Group
Cover design by Greenleaf Book Group
Cover Images: Robert Adrian Hillman/shutterstock.com; Назарій/stock.adobe.com.

Publisher's Cataloging-in-Publication data is available.

Print ISBN: 979-8-88645-201-3

eBook ISBN: 979-8-88645-202-0

To offset the number of trees consumed in the printing of our books, Greenleaf donates a portion of the proceeds from each printing to the Arbor Day Foundation. Greenleaf Book Group has replaced over 50,000 trees since 2007.

Printed in the United States of America on acid-free paper

24 25 26 27 28 29 30 31   10 9 8 7 6 5 4 3 2 1

First Edition

I dedicate this book to the thousands of patients I have had the honor and privilege to treat in my over forty years of medical practice. They have taught me to be observant, thoughtful, and compassionate. Also, to the many teachers and professors who guided me to find the way to answer questions with scientific honesty.

In Memory: Of my older brother, Martin Lonky, PhD (physics). Marty, you taught me that in the end, science is at best a living truth, based on actual data, not fear or innuendo. You were my role model for so many years, and I honor you with this dedication. I know you're still proving and disproving hypotheses with God.

Medical Disclaimer for
Outsmarting Obesity

The information provided in this book is intended for general informational purposes only. It is not a substitute for professional medical advice, diagnosis, or treatment. Always seek the advice of your physician or other qualified health provider for any questions you may have regarding a medical condition.

This book's content is based on the author's research and experience. While every effort has been made to ensure its accuracy and completeness, no guarantee is made that the information is free of errors or omissions. The author and publisher are not responsible for any actions taken or not taken based on the information provided in this book.

Obesity is a complex medical condition that requires individualized assessment and treatment. The strategies and recommendations in this book may not be suitable for everyone, and it is essential to consult with a healthcare professional before making any significant changes to your diet, exercise routine, or medical treatment.

The author and publisher do not endorse or promote any specific products, treatments, or services mentioned in this book. Any references to specific products or services are for informational purposes only and should not be considered endorsements. In no event shall the author or publisher be liable for any damages arising from the use of this book, its content, or any related materials. The reader assumes full responsibility for their actions and decisions related to their health.

By reading this book, you acknowledge and agree to the terms of this medical disclaimer. If you do not agree with these terms, you should not use this book or its information as a basis for any health-related decisions. Always consult with a qualified healthcare professional for personalized medical advice and guidance.

Contents

Foreword

America is a role model for how freedom can lead to unprecedented prosperity and opportunity.

Unfortunately, the great freedom of choice we have as individuals has led to an unprecedented increase in poor health and obesity, from kids to seniors. Indeed, poor health and obesity appear to be two of America's top growth sectors, even though the US spends more on healthcare than any other industrialized nation.

Some years ago, I read an American Heart Association report stating that heart disease will increase by approximately 10 percent by 2030 and probably even more because of soaring diabetes and obesity. Thus, in the next twenty years, over 40 percent of the population may have cardiovascular disease, increasing medical costs to cover treatments for hypertension, arterial disease, heart failure, and stroke.

Such numbers speak volumes about an entire nation out of sync with nature and common sense. During my nearly four decades of practicing cardiology and integrative medicine, I regularly saw out-of-sync patients in real cardiovascular trouble. In addition, many of them had severe weight problems, exacerbating their disease status.

In 1952, at the American Public Health Association's annual meeting, the director of New York's Bureau of Nutrition, Norman Jolliffe, warned doctors of "a new plague, although an old disease, [that had] arisen to smite us." He spoke of the 25 to 30 percent of Americans who were overweight or obese.

In retrospect, a 25–30 percent overweight/obesity rate seems benign. However, the current circumstances are significantly worse. Weight gain is a superplague. About 72 percent of adult Americans are overweight or obese, and one-third of youngsters are too heavy.

Our burgeoning waistlines bode poorly for our life quality and quantity. The too-heavy patients I encountered over the years were eating themselves into oblivion with convenient, calorie-dense processed food; they didn't exercise or address their stress.

Obesity costs our country dearly. It predisposes people to depression, diabetes, cancer, hypertension, heart disease, and premature death. In addition, obesity-related illnesses contribute to more lost workdays than all other chronic ailments combined and drive up pharmaceutical and hospital expenditures for palliating preventable but untreatable degenerative diseases.

Experts blame this mess on the dissolution of family and social cohesiveness; the 24/7 onslaught of food advertising and marketing; a shift away from quality, freshly prepared meals to convenient, calorie-dense processed foods; and, of course, an increasingly sedentary lifestyle.

Some people have suggested the government take a more prominent role in solving our weight problems. But promoting public awareness about better health and nutritional habits and encouraging physical exercise hasn't stopped the overweight jugger-naut. Moreover, the government has enacted policies that perpetuate food industry distortions—from insane farm bill subsidies that pay farmers not to grow crops and drive up the cost of fresh produce to well-intentioned but misguided food pyramids. Besides, I don't think it is the government's role to tell farmers what to farm and the eating public what to eat.

Americans turn in record numbers to magic cures, pills, sup-plements, drinks, diet plans, and know-it-all gurus, spending an estimated $76 billion annually on these and other new and bet-ter ways to lose weight. But unfortunately, the choices are endless, bewildering, and often contradictory.

We can't look to the food industry for salvation, either. The sector has to watch its bottom line. Its business strategy is to lure hun-gry, bargain-conscious consumers with a combination of tempting images, misleading claims (such as low fat, no fat, gluten-free, no cholesterol), cheap look-and-taste-enhancing additives, slick pack-aging, and plenty of sugar and salt.

While our nutrition knowledge has advanced considerably, the accumulated wisdom hasn't resulted in any consensus on what makes up a healthy diet.

On the cardiology front, an international group of researchers recently concluded that there was no objective evidence that sat-urated fat consumption increases the risk of cardiovascular events like heart attacks—a point I've made for years.

As an integrative medicine doctor, I recommended lifestyle changes to improve patients' cardiovascular health and facilitate weight loss. Such recommendations, along with encouragement, helped many patients improve their health. Those who came to me for advice were probably more inclined to overhaul their lifestyle than non-cardiac patients. They were motivated because of the apparent risks of their cardiovascular condition. Still, such advice often fell on deaf ears, and I couldn't do much to help them.

When my colleague Dr. Stewart Lonky approached me about the ideas behind the book you're about to read, I was immediately interested. I have always tried to keep an open mind regarding health, and here was a perspective from an esteemed colleague that appeared to represent a missing link. There's always more to know, even for a physician!

Even though he is a pulmonologist by training, Dr. Lonky is a world-class researcher who has long cared for patients with morbid obesity. After almost four decades of treating the heaviest patients, he has learned two critical lessons.

There is no single cause of obesity.

In treating people once they become obese, we're sometimes dealing with an underlying disease that was present even before birth.

It long ago dawned on Dr. Lonky that Western medicine treats obesity like most chronic illnesses—reactively treating or palliating symptoms without first trying to understand or correct the root causes. Long ago, I came to that same conclusion regarding cardiovascular disease.

Dr. Lonky realized he could only make a difference in his patients' lives by first acknowledging a bitter truth: the medical establishment wasn't interested in addressing obesity's root causes. Instead, they spent time, money, and resources treating obesity's symptoms. Unfortunately, this approach is akin to treating a fever without addressing the fever's cause.

Intuitively, Dr. Lonky knew the overly simplistic "eat less, exercise more" mantra for weight loss couldn't explain the alarming rise in weight problems for both young and old. And he thought the medical system didn't understand why we collectively have gained so much weight.

Dr. Lonky felt it was a waste to spend his time treating symptoms. Instead, to make a real difference in his patients' lives, he would need to understand obesity's root causes. Only then would a potential solution emerge.

Finding obesity's true causes wouldn't be a simple task. Contrary to what many have written or what you may have read, obesity isn't simply a disease of being overweight. Indeed, weight isn't the problem. Although it causes problems, weight is merely a symptom of living in a world that predisposes us to weight gain.

In *Outsmarting Obesity*, you will read an essential, well-written revelation about a new angle for understanding and perhaps preventing obesity. By the end of the book, you will understand more and have new insights and actionable ideas.

You will learn why our attempts to treat and prevent obesity often fail. But, most importantly, you will learn new strategies for reversing and preventing this affliction of modern living.

The information offered in the pages of this book rises to the level of a missing link. It's a wake-up call for all of us to change our lives.

—Stephen Sinatra, MD

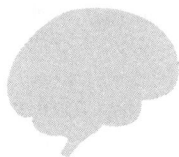

Why We Are Not Outsmarting Obesity

A Cautionary Tale

"I'm trying. I want to feel better," says Beatrice, staring up at me from the hospital bed that's been her home for the better part of a month.

Beatrice, age forty-two, stands five feet four with a weight steadily approaching 400 pounds. She once held a senior managerial level job in the human resources department of a leading financial company, a position that demanded tact, efficiency, and organization—qualities she exudes. That was 125 pounds ago.

She's just too sick these days to hold down a regular job. She has a small but close circle of family and friends who would do anything for her. Beatrice has a clear sense of who she is but more than a few illusions of who she's not. Her long brown hair is pulled back in a ponytail, revealing a classic oval face and a fair complexion.

We talk about her family and volunteer work at her church, and she tears up several times during the conversation, especially when she talks about her family's struggles with weight. "Everybody in my family is sick and fat. I don't want to go that way," Beatrice confides, her body visibly shaking as she contemplates what might be in store.

Beatrice's concerns about her family's weight problems remind me of other patients—expectant mothers who are obese and—who obsessively worry about how their excess weight might affect their unborn children. And as we'll learn later in this book, they have reason for concern.

As Beatrice and I talk further, she describes the humiliation of buying two seats and asking for a seatbelt extender on a plane, and not going to the movies because the seats are too narrow. She recalls the time she signed up for a dating service, put down as body type "a few extra pounds," got a few responses, and then, opting for honesty, changed it to "large." After that, she got none.

High blood pressure, varicose veins, pain, edema in her feet and ankles, type 2 diabetes, hypertension, gout, depression, and skin infections ravage Beatrice's body—all the downstream effects of excessive weight.

"You take control for a while," she says, "then you fail again, and you're more depressed than ever."

It's a sad situation. Beatrice's body fills the oversized hospital bed; railings lined with heavy padding minimize skin chafing and prevent her massive body from spilling out. Unfortunately, Beatrice is so large that she cannot transfer herself from the bed to a chair without help. Once seated in the chair, nurses fasten a safety strap around her torso to prevent her from falling.

As the nurses leave the room, I overhear them talking about Beatrice. "Would you look at her? I don't know how this woman got so big," whispers one nurse, who, it so happens, is six months pregnant with her first child. "I'd never let that happen to my baby or me," she adds, her voice trailing off as the door closes.

I don't think Beatrice overheard their unkind remarks. She's too consumed with her plight to notice much else. I empathize with Beatrice. She's in trouble. Even the most minor cut can quickly become a festering, limb-threatening wound in her highly compromised state.

I'm not one to gloss over problems, and I don't pull any punches with my patients. However, I'm also leery of throwing a match on gasoline. Obese patients already feel awful about themselves. Society stereotypes them as lazy, incompetent, unattractive, and lacking willpower. They're unfairly blamed for their excess weight, compounding their problems.

We talk more about her most pressing medical issues. One is right heart failure (RHF), a comparatively rare but serious condition where the right ventricle loses its pumping function, causing blood to seep into other body areas and producing congestion. It's mainly caused by low oxygen levels, and right heart failure is the reason Beatrice first became my patient.

We check off each of Beatrice's ailments—but I'm furrowing my brow through much of the conversation. Each of Beatrice's various pains and infinite medical problems end and begin with her weight. I can temporarily ease Beatrice's pain with pills, control her infections with antibiotics, and even supplement her low oxygen levels. Still, obesity complicates any treatment and exacerbates her legion of maladies. I leave Beatrice's room feeling helpless, frustrated by the circumstances that brought her to this point.

Why do we get stuck?

Physicians wear many hats. We're not here only to diagnose and treat medical problems, but also to determine and address the causes of underlying illnesses. Some patients are innocent victims saddled with diseases that result from a family member's choices and behaviors, lousy genetics, hazardous conditions at work, or just plain old bad luck. Others don't garner reflexive empathy; they fall uncomfortably into the "blame the victim" category. Pronouncing smokers as the victims of their own vice comes most immediately to mind, but people like Beatrice are right there too. "How about a little self-control," I heard the pregnant nurse mumble under her breath after she helped Beatrice to the bathroom. We rarely hear heart disease patients taken to task for their condition, though we could prevent up to 90 percent of heart disease cases by modifying diet and lifestyle factors.

Obesity is in a category all its own. Even today, too many people still view obesity only as a behavior-based disease. Obesity is a choice, they say. After all, no one is forcing us to down doughnuts at gunpoint.

Here's the problem with that line of reasoning: Obesity is never about just one thing. When over 100 million people in one country alone suffer from the same life-threatening illness, there's more than one root cause!

Origins Known and Unknown

How did we arrive here, exactly? How do we explain the obesity epidemic? Ask ten people, and you'll get twenty explanations. In 1960, when President-elect John F. Kennedy openly ruminated about the nation's declining fitness levels in an essay for *Sports Illustrated* titled "The Soft American," roughly 45 percent of adults were overweight, including 13 percent classified as obese.[1] Today, about 43 percent of Americans are obese, and our daily calorie consumption hovers at 2,700, about 500 calories over where it was forty years ago.[2] We now rank as the world's fattest developed nation, ahead of Australia and New Zealand.[3]

Whatever the cause, we can't just deal with the problem through misplaced admonitions about eating less and exercising more. Or, as former Centers for Disease Control and Prevention (CDC) Director Thomas Frieden once observed in a *New York Magazine* interview, "Exhorting people to eat less and exercise more is totally ineffectual."[4] Picking up on Dr. Frieden's point, we aren't great at making wise health choices even when we know what's best for us. Healthy eating, physical activity, avoiding tobacco and excessive alcohol consumption, and regular health screenings can prevent or limit many chronic diseases, including type 2 diabetes, cancer, and heart disease. But how many of us do these things?

Now what?

America's current approach to the obesity epidemic reminds me of the guy who tries to cure a headache by banging his head repeatedly against a brick wall. Eventually, the pain dissipates because he passes out from the cerebral concussion. That we keep trying simple, unproven solutions and getting the same result—failure— should tell us something about the well-trodden path on which we now find ourselves.

No one seems to know all the reasons for the substantial global obesity numbers, which recently surpassed 1 billion people. What I think has happened is that by considering the most obvious variables, we've overlooked some of the most critical facts. All the talk about empty calories, too much channel surfing, and too little physical activity can't explain the ballooning of a particular population segment that doesn't go to the movies, watch television, and order takeout: babies. Indeed, the prevalence of obese infants under six months has risen 73 percent since 1980.[5] So yes, something else is at work.

Our Toxic Burden

The search for the non-obvious explanation has led to an all-too-familiar villain: toxic compounds. Just look around. They're in the food you eat, the water you drink, the air you breathe, and the products that touch your skin. Each of us carries a secret stash of toxic compounds acquired during the everyday business of living. Today, we refer to these chemicals as *obesogens* because they appear to disrupt the hormonal mechanisms regulating body weight, even in those following a reduced-calorie diet and intense exercise regimen.

Toxic compounds aren't the sole reason we're fat. However, they're arguably the obesity epidemic's most important and overlooked cause and partially explain why current interventions fall flat.

How Our Experiences Affect Our Children

Science frequently characterizes the intricacies of inherited diseases within the context of the age-old "nature versus nurture" debate, an enduring concept that paints a vivid picture of a relentless struggle between the deterministic genetic sequences encoded in our DNA and our environment's dynamic, ever-evolving influences. This is an oversimplified dichotomy, but it nevertheless provides a foundation for exploring the intricate interplay between genetic predisposition and external influences. It is not merely a matter of nature versus nurture, but a complex interweaving of both elements, where genes set the stage and environmental factors choreograph the performance.

Nevertheless, in the face of this intricate dance between nature and nurture, society often seeks more straightforward solutions to health-related issues. This desire for simplicity leads many to navigate the labyrinthine landscape of books, programs, supplements, pills, and an array of other products, all of which promise an easily accessible path to a leaner and healthier existence. Every year, we witness a deluge of new diet plans, each touting a revolutionary and improved method for shedding excess weight. It seems like a relentless parade of inventive strategies, each vying for our attention and trust.

The irony inherent in this continuous stream of diet inventors and their promises lies in the question: What would these diet creators have to invent if any of their approaches truly worked? The relentless innovation and marketing of new diet plans appear to be a testament to the persistent struggle of millions to find a simple and effective solution to weight management. In a world inundated with many options, it becomes increasingly clear that a one-size-fits-all approach to health and weight management remains elusive.

Indeed, the chances of a person sticking with any regimen are low, while the likelihood of falling off the wagon and regaining weight with interest is relatively high. The esteemed *New England Journal of Medicine* found that two-thirds of dieters return to baseline within a year, and 95 percent regain their lost weight within five years.[6]

In our hyperconnected, instant-information world, advice once accessible only to the rich and famous is now available to everyone. Perhaps the problem is that most advice misses the mark and is impossible for many people to follow, especially the heaviest among us.

In medicine, untangling the correlation and causation web is complex, and factors frequently overlap in ways that makes it easy to mistake them. For instance, it is often the case that autism and autism spectrum disorders are diagnosed during the same period when children receive multiple vaccinations. Nevertheless, it's crucial to emphasize that there is no established link between vaccines and autism; the majority of available evidence actually suggests otherwise. Correlation doesn't equal causation. Yet, most health professionals who treat obesity cannot recognize that there are limits to individual agency. So, just because obese people sometimes eat a poor diet does not mean that this is the only cause of their weight problems.

I can't expect my patients, many of whom are morbidly and even lethally obese—a condition I explain later in the book—to lose weight and pursue a healthier lifestyle unless they first fully understand how they got there. Likewise, telling someone to lose weight and exercise more without tangible support—which involves information and practical solutions to their problems—won't work. Every obese person who enters my office knows they're in trouble. The problem is they don't know what to do about it.

What We Can and Can't Do

For this country's estimated 142 million obese people, we can't depend on pharmaceutically inclined allopathic medicine to improve all of obesity's effects; we can't consign millions of people to a miserable life waiting for that one pill or injection that cures everything. Honestly, I'm leery of putting too much faith in pharmaceutical interventions. Obesity is a complex, multifactorial metabolic and behavioral disorder that requires people to make changes. From my experience, medicines don't make people change.

But how do we shift gears? Forming a plan of attack has proved to be anything but easy. Competing social agendas often get in the way. Is the goal to improve health, clean up the environment, or end the stigma against obese and overweight people? Should anti-obesity activists cooperate with the food industry or adopt an aggressive stance? Having more policies and regulations doesn't appear to help either. And there's a simple reason: People don't want to be told what to do. Humans crave independence and freedom. We want to call the shots and make the rules. And we especially don't want to be told what we can or can't eat, no matter how much we weigh.

AIPE

To help combat the obesity crisis, I developed a four-step, easy-to-follow plan to help anyone, whether they're obese, overweight, or just worried about their weight. I refer to this four-step plan by the first letters of each step: AIPE—Accept, Identify, Prevent, and Eliminate.

AIPE is an effective tool to help people attain and maintain better health. I aim to have every obese person adopt AIPE as a core personal value. Those who wish to avoid obesity's consequences, either for themselves or their children (already born or yet to be born), must be in tune with the teachings of AIPE. With practice, these four healthy behaviors can genuinely make a difference. Even the effects of early-life exposure to environmental toxicants and chemicals can be favorably altered and reversed. Even simply reducing exposure can have a considerable impact.

The strategies and techniques I outline in the book will help you finally take control of the behaviors, habits, foods, and ways of thinking that have kept you in the same cycles. Yes, you can eliminate those unwanted but repeated behaviors.

Talley's Take

Many obese people struggle to make healthy food choices and often feel lost in a world filled with conflicting advice.

---

continued

Thus, each chapter of *Outsmarting Obesity* includes a special bonus section with advice, tips, and nutritional guidelines from Chris Talley, MS, one of the country's leading nutrition scientists and exercise physiologists and a sought-after peak performance athletics expert. Mr. Talley's program incorporates the latest scientific research to maximize fat loss, increase metabolism, improve performance, and speed exercise recovery. These are the same tips, guidelines, and advice that have enabled hundreds of elite athletes to reach the pinnacle of their respective sports and helped some of the world's most celebrated bodies lose unwanted pounds and achieve optimal health—and they've even been known to jump-start stalled weight-loss efforts.

Mr. Talley's protocols have positively impacted the lives of thousands of people. However, it's important to note that there are no certainties in life, especially when it comes to achieving sustained weight loss. Mr. Talley firmly believes that transformative lifestyle changes can help address health issues, but it's crucial to understand that there's no one-size-fits-all solution. The results you achieve are directly linked to the effort and mindfulness you invest in your personal journey.

In that spirit, he encourages everyone to evaluate their lives and view every obstacle as an opportunity for self-reflection, personal growth, and self-improvement. Imagine the profound significance and sense of empowerment that arises when you take control of your own life.

My Role

As a physician at the forefront of the obesity epidemic, I'm not subject to conflicting agendas. I don't care about long-standing institutional and legal struggles. I'm not beholden to food and drink companies, lobbyists, farmers, agribusiness, school administrators, or nutritionists, all of whom have a stake in what, where, and when we eat. I won't lead a campaign to standardize and improve the visibility of nutritional contents on food labels, because most people who read them are already healthy and thin. The machinations of food marketers and their slick commercials don't sway me. I'm not in bed with large pharmaceutical companies and will not actively promote the latest FDA-approved miracle weight-loss drug, which will probably not work for many people. I will not advocate for a new food pyramid or plate since all the world's plates and pyramids can't account for the many variables contributing to the obesity epidemic. I have only one agenda: helping you.

To beat obesity, we need the combined efforts of people willing to fight this disease at its source and with all the tools at our disposal. Until we accept that obesity is not, and never has been, a simple problem of overeating and exercising too little or having too little willpower, tenable approaches and solutions will not emerge, and the obesity epidemic will continue.

The more we commit to comprehending the full context and range of minutiae of a problem, the greater our chances are of finding a truly effective solution.

SECTION

I

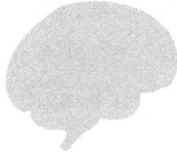

CHAPTER 1

Of Mice, Men, Monkeys, and Marmosets— The Weighty Problem of Obesity

W oody Allen isn't fat.

From what I can tell, he's never been fat. That's my observational assessment, anyway. However, that fact didn't stop the acclaimed director from obsessing over the subject. Allen transformed his plane trip literary encounters, during which he immersed himself in the pages of Dostoyevsky's "Notes from the Underground" and pored over articles from *Weight Watchers Magazine*, into a captivating essay for *The New Yorker*. "Notes from the Overfed" commenced with the stark declaration: "I am fat. I am disgustingly fat. I am the fattest human I know. I have nothing but excess poundage all over my body. My fingers are fat. My wrists are fat. My eyes are fat."[1]

While readers enjoyed Allen's poking fun at his own neuroticism and obsessive behavior by exaggerating his weight and feigning self-loathing, the real significance of Allen's essay is its 1968 publication date—a year that "changed history," proclaimed the British newspaper *The Guardian*.[2] From the emerging anti-Vietnam War and civil rights movements in the United States, to the assassinations of Martin Luther King Jr. and Robert F. Kennedy, to the iconic protests and sexual revolutions in Europe, 1968 marked a year of seismic global, social, and political shift.[3]

That year, another significant yet subtle change began to take place. At that time, the majority of the world's population maintained a healthy balance between their height and weight, and obesity was not a widespread concern. In the 1960s and 1970s only a tiny percentage of adults, around 13 percent in the United States, and an even smaller percentage of children, between 5 to 7 percent, were considered obese.[4] However, the present reality is starkly different. Obesity has evolved into a global epidemic affecting over 1 billion people and continues to rise in affluent and developing nations.

At the time of this writing, the statistics are alarming, with 21 percent of children and 43 percent of adults in the United States falling into the category of obese. Moreover, the health conditions associated with obesity, such as diabetes, cancer, heart disease, strokes, kidney failure, and dementia, are increasing at a rate that outpaces our capacity to effectively manage them. According to the World Health Organization (WHO), these health issues are projected to become the leading causes of premature death in all countries within the next decade.[5]

Also, the chronic illnesses obese people experience are far more expensive to treat than the acute, life-threatening conditions for which modern health systems are best suited. Obesity imperils individuals with decades of sickness and healthcare systems with insolvency.

Predictably, a multibillion-dollar cottage industry has arisen to address the aftereffects of our overconsumption of readily available, high-calorie, ultra-processed foods. In 2022, the weight management market in the United States achieved a market size of $73.9 billion. As forecasted by IMARC Group, a renowned market research and consulting firm, the US weight management market is projected to attain an annual valuation of $106.1 billion by 2028, reflecting a compound annual growth rate (CAGR) of 6.13 percent for the period spanning from 2023 to 2028.[6] The weight-loss industry offers a soapbox for scores of self-described experts and health and wellness influencers, all of whom will happily tell us we're too big and only with their help can our failings be addressed. The vast weight-loss industry lays the blame squarely at the feet of the 2.1 billion people who struggle with weight problems.

To some extent, they're right. We choose, repeatedly, to gorge ourselves on any number of unhealthy foods while eschewing physical activity. We always find room for an extra cookie, a handful of chips or nuts, or more French fries, but we claim we're full when presented with fresh fruit and vegetables. We reject the stairs and take the escalator. We forgo our New Year's exercise resolutions and discard our gym memberships by February, claiming we "just can't find the time" to exercise.

As our waistlines have expanded faster than the federal budget deficit, so have our tendencies toward the requisite buck-passing, shoulder shrugging, and finger pointing. From politicians to public health policy experts, no one wants to be held accountable for the nation's obesity epidemic—perhaps the United States' biggest driver of preventable chronic disease and healthcare costs.

So again, you see the "blame the patient" philosophy in public policy proposals: sky-high-deductible health plans that force obese and overweight people, who need and use more health services, to pay more out of pocket than those living at a healthy weight. There are even regulations that allow employers to charge higher health insurance premiums or impose other rewards and penalties on employees based on their health status. The Health Insurance Portability and Accountability Act (HIPAA) permits an employer to distinguish between offered benefits and benefit costs when those distinctions are not discriminatory.[7]

A Different View

On the other side of the obesity equation are people like law professor Paul Campos, who argues in his book *The Obesity Myth* that the health benefits of losing weight are mostly imaginary—a view, I might add, that most healthcare professionals do not share. Professor Campos believes the fuss we make about epidemic obesity is part of some "government-manufactured conspiracy theory, or a confabulation serving the interests of the weight-loss-pharmaceutical complex."[8]

I don't want to spend pages explaining why Professor Campos is wrong—epidemic obesity is incontrovertibly a clear, omnipresent danger. It's absurd to suggest otherwise, and it's clear he's never treated an overweight patient—most law professors haven't, to my knowledge. However, Professor Campos is correct in pointing out what I'd describe as a societal-wide moral panic about obesity. "If your child is fat, then you are a bad parent," proclaimed the headline in a column by Julia Hartley Brewer in *The Telegraph*.[9]

A recent Oklahoma State University (OSU) study suggests our health falls victim to a similar confirmation bias, as 94 percent of Americans agree that we're making ourselves fat.[10] Individual agency is obesity's favorite whipping boy. The comments range from cruel to ignorant. "No one's forcing people with weight problems to eat doughnuts or French fries." Or, "Obese people lack willpower. They're weak-minded." I know many successful people who struggle with weight problems. They don't lack willpower. Their lives are monuments to determination and personal resolve. Most are successful in every area of their lives except one.

Here's the other thing. Do you think the world's 1 billion-plus obese people, not to mention another billion who are overweight, just lost willpower and started making poor food choices simultaneously?

The Oklahoma State study raises another interesting question: Why do we keep gaining weight if we all agree that obesity is within our control? Wouldn't we simply do something about it?

Perhaps these findings show either indifference to, or more likely frustration with, weight loss. For instance, older people may view the effort needed to lose weight and extend their life span as futile. "I'm eighty-three, and now you're telling me to give up sweets. That's one of my few remaining pleasures in life. So, what's the point?" said one of my heaviest patients.

Taking Ownership

The OSU survey suggests we don't view obesity as a problem. However, I have a different take. I think we do see that a problem exists, but we don't appreciate its severity, which is the case with many chronic diseases. A collaborative survey of 1,500 adults who were classified as obese found that the overwhelming majority viewed themselves as merely overweight.[11] Today, seven in ten Americans are obese or overweight, but only 36 percent think they have a weight problem.[12]

The million-dollar question, of course, is, why don't we take obesity seriously? One problem is that obesity, while noticeable, is also insidious. As obesity expert and *Forbes* columnist Bruce Y. Lee, MD, points out, "Obesity is a global catastrophe in slow motion that moves fast enough to cause havoc but not rapidly enough for people to recognize what's happening." Of course, we see obesity happening—it's impossible to miss—but unlike a car accident or appendicitis, we don't see it as a problem until the doctor diagnoses us with atherosclerosis or metabolic syndrome and schedules a cardiac catheterization or gastric bypass surgery. "Perhaps if the global obesity epidemic moved faster, it would garner an emergency response similar to Ebola, Zika, or other infectious disease epidemics that have gripped the world in recent years," writes Dr. Lee.[13]

Dr. Lee makes a valid point. While most physicians and healthcare professionals correctly view obesity as a disease, others see it resulting from a confluence of circumstances like overeating and under-exercising—habits arising from a person's quirks, character flaws, or perceived moral shortcomings. As True Health Initiative founder and bestselling author David L. Katz, MD, once said, "Obesity has always invited the castigation of willpower and personal responsibility and the invocation of gluttony, sloth, or the combination."[14]

Forget about the Government

Can the government make a dent in the obesity epidemic? I doubt it. Government attempts to curb obesity across many countries have been ineffective and met with resistance because Big Brother's policies don't consider the emotional message they send of shame, punishment, or control.

For example, adding calorie counts to menus encouraged (and perhaps goaded) some people into making "healthier" choices while eating out. However, when confronted with the reality that a favorite frosted blueberry muffin comes packed with 400-plus calories, most of us still go for the pastry. Indeed, no matter how much calorie information the menu contains, people still choose the foods they like, not those that are supposedly healthier, according to a Carnegie Mellon research study.[15]

Interestingly, the Carnegie Mellon study found no difference between overweight/obese and healthy-weight participants in their food choice behaviors; the overweight/obese group did not choose higher calorie foods more often than the healthy weight group. And both groups underestimated the calories consumed during a meal, which supports earlier research findings.

Corpulent Critters

While we seem to have a society-wide consensus that excess body weight is the consequence of individual choice, scientists usually in the know—endocrinologists who study the biochemistry of fat and epidemiologists who study weight trends—are still in the dark about obesity's origins. However, one thing is certain: it's not simply a matter of individual choice. As former *International Journal of Obesity* editor Richard L. Atkinson said in 2005, "The previous belief of many laypeople and health professionals that obesity results from a lack of willpower and an inability to discipline eating habits is no longer defensible."[16]

Do we know if Dr. Atkinson was right? Consider this not-so-little tidbit: wild and domestic animal populations have been getting fatter for decades. According to the National Pet Obesity Survey, over 50 percent of cats and dogs—that's over 80 million pets, for anyone who's keeping score—are overweight or obese.[17] Pudgy pooches and fat felines are now so ubiquitous that there's even a National Pet Obesity Awareness Day.

Large lapdogs and comatose kitties aren't alone in the corpulent critter kingdom. In 2010, an international team of scientists led by the University of Alabama–Birmingham biostatistician

David B. Allison published findings that two dozen distinct animal populations—all cared for by or living near humans—had been rapidly fattening for the better part of three decades. In their paper, "Canaries in the Coal Mine: A Cross-Species Analysis of the Plurality of Obesity Epidemics," Dr. Allison and his colleagues found that as the American people have gotten fatter, so have America's marmosets, laboratory macaques, chimpanzees, vervet monkeys, and mice, right along with domestic dogs, cats, and urban and rural domestic and feral rats.[18]

The researchers examined records on those eight species—looking at samples collectively comprising over 20,000 individual animals from twenty-four populations living with or around humans in industrialized societies—and found that each one's average weight had increased. The marmosets gained an average of 9 percent per decade. Lab mice gained about 11 percent over the same period.

Chimps, the "canaries" most closely related to us, are also faring poorly. Between 1985 and 2005, the male and female laboratory chimps studied experienced 33.2 and 37.2 percent weight gains, respectively, leading to a fourteen-fold obesity increase. The authors note that there's no *a priori* reason that a single explanation for this weight should apply across all these populations. Still, when we see this trend across many groups, we'd be remiss not to speculate about one.

The weight spike across animal species doesn't surprise me. However, this phenomenon has little to do with overfed people tossing extra goodies to their pampered pets or leaving more calorie-laden garbage for feral cats and rodents. Such results don't explain why the weight gain is also occurring in species that human beings don't habitually pamper or have contact with, such as lab animals, which I can tell you from personal experience subsist on tightly controlled diets. Precise monitoring and measuring are the hallmarks of lab animals' lives, and it's relatively easy to rule out—or at least pinpoint—incidental human influence.

Dr. Allison and his colleagues found that lab animals gained weight over decades without significant changes to their diet or activities. So, if animals are getting heavier along with people, it can't just be that they're ordering more takeout, hitting up the local Dunkin Donuts, channel surfing, and forgoing the gym. This trend suggests the existence of a widely shared cause (or causes) beyond conscious control, contributing to obesity across many species.

Bulging Babies

Babies are also packing on the pounds just as our animal brethren are getting fatter. Statistics show that more women than ever in the US give birth to babies weighing 10 pounds or more. While there is no set figure for how much a newborn should weigh, 8 pounds 13 ounces is the general guideline for the tipping point between a healthy weight and a potentially problematic one. Alarmingly, the rate of macrosomia—the term for babies born over this tipping point—has soared in recent years.[19]

So, babies are getting fatter, but why is this happening? The most straightforward and obvious answer is that babies are getting bigger because their mothers are too. According to the latest numbers, 50 percent of childbearing-age women in the US are overweight or obese, putting their children at higher risk for weight problems.[20] This influence is so profound that the children of mothers who are obese are more likely to accumulate fat and, at some point, become obese themselves, even if they're not obese as infants.

In one study, University of Colorado School of Medicine researchers analyzed stem cells from the umbilical cords of babies born to average-weight mothers and mothers who qualified as obese. They coaxed these stem cells to develop muscle and fat cells in the lab. The resulting cells from the obese mothers had 30 percent more fat than those from normal-weight mothers, suggesting that these babies were more likely to accumulate fat.[21]

However, I don't want to focus solely on the mother's role in childhood weight gain. As with adult obesity, childhood obesity results from the dynamic interplay of genetic, behavioral, and environmental factors and dozens of broken systems affecting our health.

Weight Inequality

These hidden factors might help explain why most people gain weight gradually over many decades. The slow, inexorable increase in fat stores would suggest that we eat only a bit more each month than we burn as fuel. However, if this were the case, you'd think weight loss would be a snap. One recent model estimated that eating 30 calories more than you use per day can contribute to severe weight gain. Eating 150 calories more than you burn can lead to an extra 5 pounds over six months.[22] That's a gain of 10 pounds a year. Given what most people consume in a single day (1,500 to 2,000 calories in poorer nations; 2,500 to 4,000 in wealthy ones), 30 calories are nothing. That's half an Oreo cookie, two or three Peanut M&M's, or a tablespoon of whole-fat cottage cheese. The same holds for 150 calories. If eliminating a few bites from their daily diet were enough to prevent weight gain, people should have no trouble shedding a few pounds. Instead, as we know, the opposite is true.

Many other aspects of the global obesity epidemic don't square with the "calories in, calories out" model. In wealthy countries, we find more obesity in people with less money, education, and status.

There's an uneven excess weight distribution among the sexes, too. A study published in the journal *Social Science and Medicine* found in a sample of sixty-eight nations that for every two men there were three women who were obese.[23] So, if body weight boils down to individual food choices, why are wealth and sex factors?

The Environmental Chemicals in the Room and the Air

Back in 2005, in what many scientists point to as a seminal moment in our understanding of obesity's development, Washington State University researchers observed pregnant rats exposed to high levels of a commonly used fungicide (a toxic substance used to kill or prevent fungus growth on crops) gave birth to male offspring with low sperm counts. When these male rats matured and impregnated a female, they too gave birth to offspring with correspondingly low sperm counts. And this exposure problem didn't stop with the grandkids. It persisted through multiple generations. After years of investigation, the researchers determined that altered DNA methylation patterns in the germline were the cause.[24] So just what the heck is going on?

Layered over every strand of our cells' DNA are chemicals called methyl groups (one carbon atom surrounded by three hydrogen atoms). These methyl groups influence gene expression. DNA methylation is a commonly used, heritable epigenetic change that can cause gene expression that does not involve changes to the underlying DNA sequence. Which is to say, epigenetic modifications don't change the DNA but they do affect the gene's expression. These changes can turn a gene "on" or "off."

Epigenetic effects aren't limited to fungicides, and reproductive issues aren't the only phenotype that pops up following chemical exposure. Indeed, industrial compounds long ago entered the obesity equation. Thanks to dozens of studies, we know that bisphenol-A (or BPA), an organic compound found in many household plastics, alters lab animals' fat regulation. The same Washington State researchers who first observed the fungicide's effects on rats' reproductive health noted several fat rats following experiments on females injected with a toxic mixture of BPA and phthalates, substances used to make plastic products. Just like the tested fungicide, these compounds are endocrine disruptors—they interfere with the function of certain hormones, such as estrogen or insulin.[25]

While some environmental toxicants disrupt cell signaling, others leave specific, lasting epigenetic marks on our cells' DNA. For example, DDT, a long-banned pesticide widely used in the US in the 1970s, was found to have such effects. In one study, lab rats exposed to DDT showed methylation profiles that differed from those of rats exposed to plastic compounds. Still, the result of the DDT study mimicked that of the study involving BPA and phthalates: DDT-exposed mothers or grandmothers were of average body size. However, just one generation later, 50 percent of the rat population, male and female, were obese.[26]

Now tie these findings to obesity's dramatic rise over the last twenty-five years. Millions of women in the 1950s and 1960s were exposed to DDT. It wouldn't surprise me if these decades-old exposures had something to do with today's obesity epidemic.

It's also possible that chemical disrupters could affect people's body chemistry on longer timescales—starting, for instance, before their birth. A developing fetus is acutely sensitive to the environment into which it will be born. The nutrition it gets via the umbilical cord is a principal source of information about that environment. It's well established that pregnant women who go hungry produce offspring at a higher risk of obesity.[27] The pre-natal environment causes epigenetic changes that fine-tune a child's metabolism for a life of scarcity, preparing them to store fat. If that scarcity spell never materializes, the child's fat-storing propensity stops being an advantage. Holland's Hunger Winter famine of 1944–1945 exemplified this effect, where thousands starved to death or died of malnutrition. Yet, the 40,000 babies gestated during that year grew up to have more obesity, diabetes, and heart trouble than their compatriots who developed without the influence of war-induced starvation.[28]

While Dr. Bruce Blumberg wasn't the first to link toxic compounds to obesity, he coined a term in 2006 that would become a catch-all for environmental chemicals linked with extreme fat gain. *Obesogen* was the new term, and it defined an emerging line of scientific inquiry that challenged the weight control zeitgeist.[29] Before recent discoveries of toxicants' role in the obesity equation, many experts believed obesity resulted strictly from an energy imbalance—overeating and exercising too little. As I argue throughout this book, repeated chemical exposures—particularly those that mess with hormonal pathways—have left our bodies susceptible to obesity in the face of modern, waistline-challenging lifestyles and the failure of systems that support human health and well-being.

A Crowded Field

Beyond obesogens, there are other factors in the obesity equation, what Dr. Allison called the "roads less traveled" of obesity research.

Does light exposure increase obesity risk? In an Ohio State University study, mice exposed to constant light gained significantly more weight than those exposed to a natural light and dark cycle, even when fed the same diet. One explanation for this finding is that constant light exposure may disrupt the timing of the mice's feeding behavior and metabolic processes. In the wild, mice eat at night and rest during the day. However, constant light exposure may confuse their internal clock and disrupt their natural eating cues, leading them to eat at the wrong time of day and throwing off their metabolism.[30]

Previous research has suggested that exposure to artificial light at night can disrupt human circadian rhythms and contribute to weight gain and other health problems. The modern 24/7 lifestyle may promote obesity by encouraging us to eat at night, the time when our ancestors were asleep. For example, night shift workers gain more weight than other small demographic groups.

Is obesity contagious? Ad-36, a recognized viral agent responsible for human eye and respiratory infections, has been found to induce weight gain in various animals, including chickens, rats, mice, and monkeys. In 1992, researcher Nikhil Dhurandhar first suggested a possible link between viruses and obesity when he observed that chickens in India infected with adenovirus exhibited plumpness rather than emaciation. Dr. Dhurandhar, now a professor at the Pennington Biomedical Research Center at Louisiana State University, coined the term *infectobesity* to describe the idea of excess weight being transmitted through the spread of bugs and viruses.[31]

Of course, testing for this effect on humans would be impossible and wholly unethical. However, a study by Japanese researchers published in the journal *PLOS One* found that people infected with Ad-36 had significantly higher body mass index (BMI) than those who avoided infection.[32]

Bacteria may similarly impact weight gain. For example, the microbiome in your gut seems to affect the production of hunger hormones, such as ghrelin, which controls satiety. In addition, an unhealthy gut microbiome can increase inflammatory markers, leading to weight gain and metabolic disease. A human study first published in the *Journal of Clinical Endocrinology and Metabolism* found that overweight and obese individuals were likelier than healthy-weight folks to have elevated *Methanobrevibacter smithii* populations. These gut microorganisms digest food, assimilate nutrients, and contribute to weight gain.[33]

Paths Still Unknown

I'm not claiming, nor should anyone argue, that any of these "roads less traveled" are the primary obesity driver. They all play a role. There's no single obesity driver. It's more than believable that every one of the routes contributes, in varying degrees, to epidemic obesity.

It's simplistic to attribute obesity solely or even principally to personal responsibility. In an important book, *The Metabolic Ghetto*, Dr. Jonathan Wells, University College–London professor of anthropology and pediatric nutrition, explains obesity's origins and ubiquity. Like poverty, obesity is a "large-scale development that no one deliberately intends, but which emerges out of the millions of separate acts that together make up a whole." It is, he says, a "saga spanning many generations."[34]

In Dr. Wells's view, it is a fallacy to believe that individual choices primarily influence the global obesity epidemic. Instead, he likens it to the sentiment expressed by Tolstoy in the concluding chapters of *War and Peace*, where invisible social forces guide us much like the Earth moves through space, propelled by imperceptible physical forces. This analogy encapsulates the essence of Dr. Wells's contemporary perspective on obesity.[35]

There's more to Dr. Wells's argument, however. If you or your parents—or their parents—were undernourished, you're more likely to become obese. Obese people, when they have children, pass on changes that can predispose future generations to obesity. Like the children of underfed people, overfed children's metabolisms promote obesity. An underfed past combined with an overfed present is an obesity trap, what Dr. Wells calls a "metabolic ghetto."

Still Behind the Eight Ball

Recently, I attended a lecture during which a government official with no apparent medical training said, "It's impossible to come up with a single obesity policy because science is undecided." This statement reflects scientific ignorance. Science is always undecided, forever in a state of perpetual motion. All good scientists second-guess themselves. Expressions like "scientifically proven" are nearly oxymorons. The foundation of science is to keep the door ajar so we remain receptive to doubt—the engine of all inquiry, as the late Christopher Hitchens once suggested.

There is never a moment in science when all doubts are gone and all questions settled, which is why "waiting for settled science" is intellectual purgatory. "Settled science" is an idea created by industries that want no interference with their bottom line.

However, obesity presents us with an unusual situation because it forces us to make wise decisions about millions of people's health based on incomplete knowledge. So, of course, we must do something, using the best scientific information available, which, now, posits explanations far more complicated than human agency and overly simplistic admonitions like "calories in, calories out" and "eat less, exercise more."

The obesity era is in its infancy. We're still writing its history and will be for some time. We have some answers, but we're far from solving the puzzle. For example, suppose the obesogen theory comes to be as widely accepted as I hope and puts the human agency model in its proper context. In that case, it will be harder for the weight-loss and food industries, along with our government, to keep pushing low-calorie diets and foods that, while superficially healthy, also contain an array of substances that may contribute to weight gain.

Some folks in the weight-loss community, including Marion Nestle, an emeritus New York University professor and prolific author, advocate for stronger government regulation to help deal with the obesity epidemic. Dr. Nestle would prefer that we focus more on food production and less on food consumption. While she admits certain compounds harm our health, she says it's hard to prove they affect weight gain. Dr. Nestle told *The Atlantic*, "They might have something to do with obesity—I suppose it's possible— but why invoke complicated explanations when the evidence for calories is so strong? Let's say obesogens affect a bodyweight regulatory factor. But so, what? More than a hundred biological factors regulate weight, and they are redundant, meaning that if something goes wrong with one of them, the others fill in the deficit."[36]

It's Dr. Nestle's "so what" that troubles me. While obesity science is continually evolving, we know enough to draw more than a causal connection between toxic exposures and obesity. Meanwhile, others—food industry lobbyists, most notably—have discredited obesogen research, funding studies that produce the opposite conclusions, casting doubt.[37] BPA is a perfect example. Most studies performed by independent government and academic scientists show that BPA adversely affects human health. In contrast, food industry-funded/conducted research has failed to reveal BPA-associated hazards.[38] I'm not sure why people default to increased government regulation to help with the obesity epidemic. Indeed, this approach has been tried and has failed every time.

The other justification for government intervention—we need more nutrition information—is a non-starter. We have plenty of nutrition information. Just look at any food package or ingredient list. People aren't gaining weight, getting sick, and dying because they lack nutrition knowledge. They're getting sick and dying from the effects of being overweight and obese.

Whatever the answer, we should place less emphasis on a fragile construct like human agency and treat obesity like any other chronic illness—as a multifactorial problem for which no easy, one-size-fits-all solution exists. Unfortunately, humans habitually seek the path of least resistance. The more complex a problem, the more we desire a simple solution.

However, we should be wary of simple solutions to complex problems. There are no quick fixes for a multifactorial problem decades in the making. Accepting obesity's complexity and challenges is a step toward ridding ourselves of the idea that extreme weight gain is merely a matter of choice. Until we accept that obesity is not a simple problem, the best approaches and solutions will not emerge, and the epidemic will continue.

Talley's Take: The Scales That Bind Us

Could you imagine a professional athlete with weight problems?

Well, it happens a lot more often than you imagine.

Tennis legend Martina Navratilova famously gained 20 pounds in two weeks while subsisting on a steady diet of pancakes, cereal, and pastries.

In 2010, one of Major League Baseball's most celebrated pitchers put his uniform to the test when he tipped the scales at 315 pounds with a BMI of 36.5, thanks to boxes of Cap'n Crunch.

Before the 2015–2016 season, Miami Heat point guard Kyle Lowry, then with the Toronto Raptors, showed up to training camp weighing 210 pounds, placing him firmly in the overweight category for his six-foot frame.

Former MLB first baseman and designated hitter Prince Fielder weighed as much as 285 pounds, which is quite a lot when you consider he stands 5'10."

Tony Siragusa was one of the NFL's biggest defensive tackles, with a playing weight of 340 pounds. After retiring, he ballooned to over 400 pounds before dropping to 360. Unfortunately, Siragusa's weight loss was too little too late, as he died of a heart attack at age fifty-five. NFL offensive or defensive linemen are commonly instructed to maintain a weight of over 300 pounds to be competitive on the football field. While this may seem like an invitation for them to eat whatever they want, it's not all fun and games— maintaining such a weight can pose significant health risks.

I could go on and on. Professional athletes aren't immune to the same weight problems, including obesity, that vex the rest of us.

Indeed, one of the interesting but paradoxical observations in my work with thousands of world-class athletes is the high number living with weight problems, including obesity, despite their successful competitive sports careers.

I think the most obvious explanation for weight gain among pro athletes is simple: retirement. Unfortunately, many pro athletes stop training after retiring. They're tired, injured, or just burned out. But the abrupt halt to their training regimens doesn't improve their health.

Retirement is hard for many athletes. When their playing careers end, they're often left with bodies and routines that no longer fit their new lives—explaining why so many struggle with post-career weight gain and even body dysmorphia, a common occurrence in female athletes. If you're twenty-five years old and doing a physical activity five to six hours a day, then none of these things are on your radar.

But the paradigm shifts once an athlete calls it quits. Retired athletes left to their own devices without a team or the structures that helped mold their bodies to compete at the highest levels become just like us—easy pickings for the vicissitudes of a sedentary life. Most don't know how to keep weight off without regular physical training.

One such retired athlete, a former Philadelphia Eagles and Atlanta Falcons tackle, became one of fifteen contestants on NBC's popular reality program *The Biggest Loser*, tipping the scale at 450 pounds fourteen years after his final National Football League game.

Of course, it's not only athletes who struggle. We're in the golden age of the overweight celebrity.

In TikTok videos and Instagram posts, famous folks come clean about everything from binge eating to weight gain. And we get the chance to relate—their battles to resist the siren song of French fries or fit into a pair of skinny jeans mirror our struggles.

For many of us, seeing that the rich and famous aren't immune to the lure of junk food, despite enormous pressures and incentives to be thin, reassures us and helps us feel less alone.

Celebrity weight struggles help affirm the public's belief that the rich and famous are unique, but no different from the rest of the herd. And to some extent, that's true. We all put our pants on the same way. But celebrity weight struggles underscore that the obesity epidemic doesn't exclude famous people. Like cancer, heart disease, and dementia, no one is immune.

Celebrities breathe the same air, shop at the same food markets, and go through the same difficulties. Celebrities are not immune to the effects of endocrine-disrupting chemicals or any better at shielding themselves from unfavorable changes to their epigenomes. They own refrigerators, too, and stock them with the same tempting foods. They inhabit the same 24-hour food environment.

I don't think there's anything wrong with a famous person sharing their tale of woe. If others can relate to their experience, it might help. What we need more of, however, are celebrity weight-loss success stories. If it's true that up to 95 percent of all weight-loss efforts tank, then it's also true that up to 95 percent of celebrity weight-loss efforts fail. At my practice, Precision Food Works, where I work with some of the world's most recognized athletes, actors, and other A-listers, weight loss, particularly for those who are obese, takes time, effort, and patience. It means partnering with physicians like Dr. Lonky to ensure my clients aren't simply losing weight but are doing it safely and sustainably.

Too often, we read about some leading actress who lost 50 pounds in three months for a role and assumes that's how everyone does it. However, no one who wants to lose weight and keep it off does it this way. We have to get over our culture's instant gratification mindset. You didn't gain an extra 50 pounds in a week, so why would you expect to take it off in less time?

The good news is that most celebrities do it the right way. You just don't hear about it because slow, safe, and steady weight loss doesn't help you gain a huge TikTok following or land you a spot on a Bravo TV reality show.

And that's a shame.

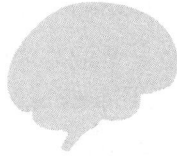

CHAPTER 2

Overweight or Undertall—
Defining Obesity

Fred, the Fat Hockey Player

At the height of his career, my patient Fred weighed 248 pounds, which for a stout, 6'3" professional hockey player isn't a big deal. Hockey players have solid and well-developed muscles, which aid their powerful and explosive strides and help them chase a puck across the ice or hit an opponent.

Plugging the numbers into the CDC's Body Mass Index (BMI) calculator, Fred's BMI comes in at 31, placing him squarely in the obese category for his height and weight. The CDC recommends a 148-to-199-pound range for a man Fred's size. My fifteen-year-old amateur hockey-playing grandson, who stands 5'11", falls into the 148-to-199-pound weight category. So how long do you think Fred would've survived in the brutal world of professional hockey at 150–160 pounds?

Fred's inclusion in the obese category highlights one of our many challenges in defining obesity. Physicians typically use BMI to measure a patient's "weight health." However, the most significant drawback of BMI is its inability to differentiate between fat and muscle. While it's not accurate to say that muscle weighs more than fat, it is denser. This density is why a cubic inch of muscle weighs more than a cubic inch of fat. Therefore, BMI will inevitably classify muscled folks like Fred as overweight or obese.

When defining obesity, nothing is as simple as it seems.

Defining Obesity

Associate Justice of the United States Supreme Court Potter Stewart was known for many great things. However, he is perhaps most renowned for his non-definition of obscenity. Justice Potter said he couldn't define obscenity, but that "I know it when I see it."[1]

Anyone trying to muster up a definition of obesity might offer a similarly curt response. We know obesity when we see it, but trying to define obesity beyond simply saying, "That guy is fat," is an altogether unique challenge.

In medicine, we must differentiate between complicated cases—those that are difficult, requiring skills such as open-heart surgery—and complex ones, those with no clear solutions, unknown and incalculable risks, or unpredictable outcomes. Obesity falls into the complex category. Obesity's complexity is why many people call it a systems disease, composed of different but interconnected components that all interact with and affect one another.[2]

Unlike simple systems with linear cause-and-effect relationships, complex systems are difficult to model——tweaking the system at one end may lead to unintended consequences elsewhere. Thus, developing system-wide interventions to reverse the obesity epidemic will prove challenging. Healthcare professionals and well-intentioned legislators may suddenly find themselves in a game of Whack-A-Mole as the system responds in unpredictable ways.

Here is an example. Prescription weight-loss drugs, which mimic the effects of the hormone glucagon-like peptide 1 (GLP) by reducing food intake and delaying gastric emptying, are all the rage recently in obesity medicine. While they offer some benefits, including significant weight loss and reduced cravings, they have drawbacks. A large clinical trial for Wegovy®—the first trial showing semaglutide's efficacy as a treatment for adult obesity—found that about 40 percent of the participants lost lean body mass, substantially higher than is ideal.[3]

Also, patients rapidly regain weight once they discontinue use of the medication. A 2022 study found that people who stopped taking Wegovy® regained two-thirds of the weight they'd lost on the drug.[4] We do not know about these medications' long-term effects on our organs, behavior, and brain function. Side effects such as nausea, vomiting, and a link to rare cases of pancreatitis still plague this newest class of drugs. The lesson here is to look skeptically at anyone claiming to have a "simple" solution to the obesity problem. If it were a simple problem, we would've solved it ages ago.

Obesity is hard to define, in part, because it's multifactorial. Here is what I mean. Science has identified hundreds of obesity-linked genes and dozens of factors that interact with these genes to cause obesity.[5] However, as I will discuss in the next chapter, genetically based obesity is rare.[6] A recent study concluded, "Multiple causative and contributory factors may be present in any individual. Such factors vary inter-individually, leading to a distinct expression of obesity in each individual."[7]

Real estate agents are fond of saying, "Location is everything." The same holds for experts who define obesity by body fat distribution. In a short paper published in 1947, Jean Vague, a French professor from the University of Marseille, commented that obesity's many metabolic complications correlate more with the regional fat distribution than with how much fat a person has. Where the fat is located matters most according to this theory.

Dr. Vague described two large body shapes: *android obesity*, an apple shape representing upper body fat accumulation; and *gynoid obesity*, the infamous pear shape that describes fat accumulation around the hips and thighs. The latter is more common among women than men. In a second paper published ten years later, Dr. Vague wrote that android obesity "not only is associated with premature atherosclerosis and diabetes, but it is also the usual cause of diabetes in the adult in 80 to 90 percent of the cases."[8] Dr. Vague's papers have led some to consider hip and waist circumference a better measure than BMI for defining obesity. However, this measurement has not been universally adopted. We can say that the waist-to-hip ratio (a metric the World Health Organization uses) could measure abdominal obesity.

It gets increasingly murky as we try to unravel an actual definition of obesity that is both scientifically accurate and understandable. We first need that definition; only then can we do something.

The Scientific Challenges: Finding a Cause

Genetic, environmental, sociocultural, physiological, medical, behavioral, and epigenetic factors all influence the pathogenesis of obesity:

- To date, over 140 genetic chromosomal regions have been identified that are related to obesity. These regions contain a variety of genes and genetic variants that contribute to obesity's development in different ways. For example, some variants heighten obesity risk by increasing appetite and food intake, while others influence energy expenditure and physical activity levels.[9]

- BMI and obesity-associated gene expression occur in the central nervous system. Obesity genes probably act within the hypothalamus, a structure deep in our brain that impacts neural circuits that reward us for our decisions and the learning we gain from our experiences and memories.[10]

- Epigenetic factors can enhance adult obesity risk. Epigenetic changes refer to changes that occur on a gene's surface that are frequently transmitted to future generations, a topic I discuss in subsequent chapters.

- Disrupted sleep patterns, mental stress, environmental exposures, neurologic dysfunction, and viral infections also contribute to obesity.

- Interactions among many diseases can lead to excessive weight gain.

- Gut microbiota, the bacteria in our intestines, can also play a role in promoting obesity. According to the Obesity Medicine Association's Obesity Algorithm, "pro-inflammatory signals generated in response to the fatty sugars (lipopolysaccharides) that make up bacterial cell walls may affect neurobehavioral brain centers and impair the functioning of fat cells causing adiposopathy [a fancy word for a sick fat cell] and an increased risk for metabolic disease."[11]

Here's what we know regarding a consensus on body fat and what makes up obesity: Strangely enough, there isn't one. To understand why there is no consensus, one only needs to look at the latest conflicting obesity research. Interpreting the results can be bewildering and frustrating, particularly when leading experts disagree on fundamental questions, such as "Can you be healthy at any size?"

Another problem with defining obesity is that there aren't good metrics to say someone is obese. For example, a normal-weight patient asked me recently if she could be obese. My short answer was, "Yes, if you're at a healthy weight but your body fat percentage is over a certain threshold, you may have obesity—specifically a condition known as normal-weight obesity." Unfortunately, my answer only added to her confusion. Normal-weight obesity means you may have the same serious health risks as someone with obesity, including heart disease, metabolic syndrome, and type 2 diabetes, even if you're not overweight.

So, if there's no consensus definition of obesity, then the only alternative is to come up with a description that is both accurate and reflects the severity of the health problems that come with it.

What about BMI?

At some point—whether at the doctor, at the gym, or online—all of us have probably encountered Body Mass Index (BMI), a mathematical formula devised in the 1830s to determine whether you're a healthy weight for your height.[12] According to BMI metrics, you're of normal weight if your BMI falls between 18.5 and 24 and overweight if it's between 25 and 30. Having a BMI of 30 or more is defined as being obese. However, as I mentioned earlier, BMI is flawed because it doesn't measure body fat. Also, BMI doesn't account for other factors affecting body weight, including muscle mass, bone density, overall body composition, age, or racial and sex differences. So it's possible to have a normal BMI but have a body fat percentage high enough to increase health risks.

BMI's shortcomings highlight the need for accurate, practical, and affordable tools and techniques to measure fat and skeletal muscle and biomarkers that can better predict disease and mortality risks. Such tools could help us determine a person's ideal weight, accounting for age, sex, genetics, fitness, pre-existing diseases, novel blood markers, and the metabolic parameters obesity alters. Unfortunately, no such metrics have emerged. Since every single Electronic Medical Record (EMR) system has a built-in BMI calculation, doctors default to that measurement.

But now you know that's not the complete story.

The Pros and Cons of Using BMI

While BMI can provide some helpful information, it has limitations and should be considered just one of many factors in assessing a person's health. Here are some of the pros and cons of using BMI as a tool for health assessment.

Pros:

- Simplicity: BMI is easy to calculate using a person's weight and height, making it a quick and accessible tool for health professionals and individuals.

- Population-level insights: In large populations, BMI is useful for studying and comparing the prevalence of people who are overweight or obese.

- Risk assessment: In some cases, a high BMI can be an indicator of increased risk for certain health conditions, such as heart disease, type 2 diabetes, and some types of cancer.

continued

Cons:

- Lack of precision: BMI does not consider factors like muscle mass, bone density, and fat distribution, which can vary significantly among individuals. As a result, it may not accurately assess an individual's health.

- Doesn't differentiate between fat and muscle: A person with a high BMI might have a high percentage of muscle and low body fat, while another person with the same BMI could have a high percentage of body fat and low muscle. This can lead to misleading health assessments.

- Ignores other essential factors: BMI does not consider other important factors that impact health, such as diet, physical activity, overall body composition, genetics, and specific medical conditions.

- Can stigmatize individuals: Relying solely on BMI for health assessment can lead to the stigmatization of people who may have a healthy body composition but fall into the overweight or obese BMI categories.

- Not suitable for all populations: BMI was developed based on data from predominantly white populations and may not be as accurate for assessing the health of individuals from diverse racial and ethnic backgrounds.

To be clear, BMI is a useful tool for population-level assessments and a rough indicator of potential health risks associated with excess body weight. However, it has significant limitations when applied to individual health assessments. Health professionals often use a combination of measures, including waist circumference, body fat percentage, and other health indicators, to better understand a person's health status. It's important to recognize that BMI is just one piece of the puzzle and should be interpreted in the context of other health-related factors.

Adiposity, Adipokines, and Adiposopathy— Why is this fat unlike all other fats?

We regard obesity as a far-reaching public health issue because of its connection to many life-threatening health problems. However, it's also true that excess fat accumulation doesn't affect everyone the same way. In some people, obesity increases cardiovascular disease and dementia risk. In others, it does not. So, what's the missing link? How about "sick fat," a condition known in medical circles as adiposopathy?

In this book, I define obesity many times. For example, the Obesity Medicine Association calls obesity a "chronic, relapsing, multifactorial neurobehavioral disease" with a corresponding rise in "adipose tissue dysfunction, resulting in adverse metabolic and biomechanical effects and negative psychosocial consequences."[13] That's not only a mouthful but also a complicated definition. Yet, it's important because it points out that adipose tissue dysfunction is synonymous with adiposopathy. So, I want to examine adipose tissue's role in adiposopathy and its impact on metabolic health.

Subcutaneous fat, found just beneath the skin, might be considered unattractive by some, but it is relatively benign. On the other hand, fat surrounding internal organs, often referred to as visceral fat, elevates the risk of metabolic irregularities. Research suggests that people with excess visceral fat have a higher risk of diabetes, lipid disorders, and cardiovascular disease than those with less visceral fat.[14]

The discovery of a pathological significance to adipose tissue's location led to new research on its role. Adipose tissue is a metabolically dynamic organ vital in energy storage and release. However, it's also a vibrant and critical endocrine organ capable of synthesizing several biologically active compounds that regulate metabolic homeostasis. It is fatty tissue's endocrine function that we will concern ourselves with here.

What does adipose tissue actually do?

Perhaps the best place to start is with fat itself. It's there for a reason, right?

Fat makes hormones. Through these hormones' actions, adipose tissue regulates glucose, cholesterol, and sex hormone metabolism. Adipocytes (fat cells) even secrete hormones that tell us when we're hungry and full. The hormones our fat tissue makes regulate various bodily functions. Examples include:

- Aromatase, which is involved in sex hormone metabolism (it converts androgens into estrogens)

- TNF alpha, IL-6, and leptin, which are collectively termed "cytokines" and involved in sending messages between cells

- Plasminogen activator inhibitor-1, which is involved in blood clotting

- Angiotensin, responsible for constricting blood vessels and aiding in the regulation of blood pressure and the body's fluid equilibrium

- Adiponectin, which improves the body's insulin sensitivity and helps protect against developing type 2 diabetes

- Lipoprotein lipase and apolipoprotein E, which play essential roles in both storing and breaking down fats to release energy[15]

Like every other bodily organ, adipose tissue may become diseased. Consequently, adiposopathy was defined and used to describe adipose tissue dysfunction, including fat accumulation (adiposity). It also means that the hormones I just mentioned don't function properly. Hence, the term "sick fat."

From Healthy to Sick Fat Cells

Scientists believed for many years that we were born with a certain number of fat cells and that new cell production stopped early in life. Instead, we now know fat cell numbers stay relatively constant (even after marked weight loss), showing that childhood and adolescence set our fat cell count. Of course, we replace old and dying fat cells, and research suggests that up to 10 percent of fat cells renew every year.[16]

When we overeat, adipose tissue responds by recruiting more fat cells. This occurrence is known as hyperplasia, a process characterized by the multiplication of fat cells, allowing adipose tissue to accumulate excess energy as fat. However, if too few new cells heed adipose tissue's cry, the existing adipocytes take up the slack by getting bigger, a phenomenon called hypertrophy. Unfortunately, hypertrophy leads to fat cell dysfunction, which provokes abnormal endocrine and immune responses, eventually leading to the sort of metabolic abnormalities we typically see in sick fat. For example, one study showed that type 2 diabetes patients had a lower total adipocyte number but that their existing fat cells were bigger, independent of body weight.[17]

In obesity, adipocyte hypertrophy is frequently associated with an inflammatory response that leads to the development of insulin resistance in adipose tissue. However, recent data show that even without an inflammatory reaction, hypertrophic fat cells are insulin resistant, suggesting that adipocyte hypertrophy may play a crucial role in causing insulin resistance in obese people.[18]

The adipocyte hypertrophy and insulin resistance relationship is significant because insulin resistance substantially increases cardiovascular disease, type 2 diabetes, high blood pressure, stroke, nonalcoholic fatty liver disease, polycystic ovary syndrome, and cancer risk.

There is a lot of ongoing speculation about why large adipocytes become sick. One theory is that large adipocytes are likelier to suffer from hypoxia because oxygen can't diffuse into such a large cell. Another view is that there is significant inflammation in the tissue surrounding these cells due to an increased production of inflammation-related proteins called adipokines. I believe both are true, and some data show that hypoxia worsens this inflammatory response—we have hypoxic adipose tissue from animal models that bears this out.

Adipokines

You might have heard the phrase "cytokine storm" during the height of the COVID-19 pandemic. Many COVID-19 complications result from a condition known as cytokine release syndrome (CRS) or a cytokine storm. CRS happens when a stimulus (infection or other) triggers the immune system to flood your bloodstream with inflammatory proteins called cytokines. They can kill tissue and damage organs.

However, not all cytokines are harmful. A broad range of cells produce cytokines and play a significant role in keeping us healthy. To illustrate, fatty tissue produces a class of cytokines known as adipokines. These adipokines serve as messengers facilitating communication between adipose tissue and the immune, endocrine, and cardiovascular systems. This unique function leads us to categorize adipose tissue as an endocrine organ because it releases substances that govern and oversee the functioning of other cells and organs.

Fat Talking: Does adipose tissue communicate with other organs?

Is there more to that beer gut than meets the eye?

It seems that way. Fat tissue is so smart that it can communicate with other organs, sending out tiny molecules controlling gene activity in other body parts. This novel cell-to-cell communication highway shows that fat is truly an endocrine organ that plays a significant role in regulating metabolism. It also opens the door to new treatment options for obesity, diabetes, and other metabolic diseases.

While scientists understand the relationship between fat and disease, they don't fully grasp how fat tissue affects distant organs and their functions. Long ago, scientists identified hormones secreted by fat, such as leptin, that signal the brain to regulate eating. However, in 2017 they looked at another messenger— tiny bits of genetic material called microRNAs or miRNAs.[19]

MiRNAs help control gene expression and protein production throughout the body. But miRNAs venture out

continued

independently, traveling freely through the bloodstream, bundled into tiny packets called exomes—regions of the genome that encode proteins. Exomes make up just 1–2 percent of the genome but contain approximately 85 percent of disease-causing variants. High miRNA levels have been associated with obesity, diabetes, cancer, and cardiovascular disease.[20, 21]

Scientists studied genetically engineered mice whose fat cells lacked a critical miRNA-processing enzyme to understand how miRNAs function in fat. These rodents had less fat tissue and couldn't process glucose as effectively as non-engineered mice. However, they also had low circulating miRNA levels overall.

By transplanting fat from normal-weight mice, the researchers restored the modified mice's previously low miRNA levels. In addition, these transplants of "brown fat"—specialized energy-burning fat that regulates temperature—helped restore glucose processing in the genetically modified mice, whereas "white fat"—energy-storing fat—transplants did not.[22]

In another study, mice with low miRNA production were found to have abnormalities in other organs, such as the heart and liver. Looking at the mechanism for this, researchers discovered that miRNA could bind to liver cells and regulate the expression or activity of specific genes in the liver. Their findings confirmed that fat tissue, through exosomes, can communicate with the liver and regulate gene expression. These data provide insights into new pathways of tissue communication that disease states alter. If researchers can figure out how to engineer exomes to target specific cell types, they might one day use the vesicles to deliver drugs and other therapies.[23]

Although adipokines play a significant role in normal bodily processes, they likely contribute to several illnesses, including obesity, type 2 diabetes, and cardiovascular disease. In addition, adipokines' role in healthy energy metabolism and their effect on appetite and eating behavior predictably influence body weight.[24]

Adiponectin, leptin, and resistin are the most studied adipokines. So how do they impact our weight?

Obesity and visceral obesity are associated with a low plasma concentration of adiponectin. Thus, it's believed that adiponectin deficiency may play a role in obesity and the adverse metabolic consequences of visceral fat accumulation.

Adipocytes also synthesize leptin, an amino acid hormone. Leptin production correlates with fatty tissue amounts, explaining why obese folks produce more leptin than people with normal body weight. Leptin regulates energy intake and eating behavior through receptors in the brain by providing feedback information about the status of energy reserves. In other words, fatty tissue uses leptin to communicate with the hypothalamus. The signals can be twofold.

First, increased leptin production signals anorexigenesis, indicating satiety (a sense of fullness) and more than enough energy to burn. However, decreased leptin production signals orexigenesis, which communicates hunger and the need to increase energy stores. Orexigenic neurons stimulate eating; anorexigenic neurons suppress appetite.

Although leptin reduces appetite, obesity is associated with higher circulating leptin concentrations.[25] Since it was subsequently shown that obese individuals are often leptin resistant, this apparent contradiction makes sense. In obesity, the leptin isn't working at the cellular level, but the adipocyte doesn't know that, so it keeps making more leptin. This phenomenon is similar to insulin resistance in type 2 diabetes, where the pancreas produces insulin initially, but the body's cells don't respond. So, the elevated leptin in obesity fails to control hunger and reduce appetite. There is leptin there, but the brain has muted the message.

Scientists believe that normal adipokine production and secretion are affected when adipose tissue becomes sick. Diseased adipose tissue shows signs of dysregulated adipokine production.[26] In obesity, increased inflammatory mediators, such as IL-6, TNF-alfa, and reduced adiponectin output may promote further inflammation and insulin resistance. Hence, abnormal or inappropriate adipokine secretion may be an essential link between sick fat and the metabolic abnormalities associated with obesity, type 2 diabetes, and cardiovascular disease.[27]

So, obesity promotes systemic inflammation, and inflammation promotes obesity. This inflammatory state results in changes in insulin sensitivity, promoting the development of diabetes. Therefore, it looks like obesity is, in and of itself, an inflammatory disease. In a sense, when there is obesity, there is a constant inflammatory state in our bodies. Therefore, it's hard not to see obesity as a disease.

Inflammation: The Lynchpin

The discovery of systematic inflammation as an essential health factor is relatively recent, and researchers are still working to understand the mechanisms and implications. Exactly how obesity triggers inflammation is uncertain, but the inflammation process seems to be a type of immune response. Scientists believe that a macronutrient excess in fat tissues stimulates the release of inflammatory mediators such as tumor necrosis factor and interleukin 6, which reduce adiponectin production, predisposing the tissue to a pro-inflammatory state and increasing oxidative stress. Remember that adiponectin, a fat-derived hormone, protects against insulin resistance/diabetes, obesity, and atherosclerosis.[28, 29]

Obesity-induced inflammation represents a focused and rapid response to an injury site or the innate immune system responsible for fighting new threats. An infection is one such threat, but unlike the defensive or acute inflammatory response following an infection, obesity-induced inflammation is chronic and doesn't easily resolve.

In this case, fat cells and the tissue surrounding them maintain the injury and begin the inflammatory process, disrupting metabolic homeostasis. The process goes as follows:

- The immune system recognizes the injury and sends an array of inflammatory cytokines.

- These cytokines travel to adipose cells, the liver, the pancreas, and sometimes the brain and muscle tissues.

- Some experimental data show other immune cells, such as natural killer cells (a type of T cell) and macrophages, are activated.

- Changes appear in the T cell population within fatty tissue. However, there seems to be a decrease in regulatory T cells, which would keep this response in check.[30]

There is an association between increased weight gain and increased inflammation because more weight often means more inflammation. Conversely, weight loss translates to less inflammation.

Gut inflammation may also be a contributing factor and can lead to weight gain. For this reason, many dietary interventions focus on prebiotics and probiotics. In addition, eating a balanced diet with lots of fresh vegetables enhances gut health.

A Smarter Definition of Obesity: An Inflammatory Disease

As I have said earlier, people define obesity using a metric such as BMI, body weight alone, or even the hip and waist circumference ratio. Still, once we're given the number, we know nothing about obesity. Outside of saying something like "Let's lose weight," there isn't anything about those definitions of obesity that bring us any closer to understanding this disease.

But now we have a common factor—inflammation. So, by insisting on having this in the definition, we are a lot closer to identifying obesity's causes. With that, what kinds of new approaches could we find to manage and reverse a troubling trend—the increasing percentage of the public with obesity?

Does obesity fit the strict definition of a disease? According to *Mosby's Dictionary of Medicine, Nursing & Health Professions*, a disease is:

1. A condition of abnormal vital function involving any structure, part, or system of an organism;

2. A specific illness or disorder characterized by recognizable signs and symptoms attributable to heredity, infection, diet, or environment.[31]

Answer? Obesity fits.

Others have grappled with this question before. We're now nearly nine years removed from the American Medical Association's

(AMA) House of Delegates' formal declaration of obesity *as a disease state requiring treatment and prevention efforts*.[32] So, in theory, this welcome news meant that obesity rates would drop, and society would no longer view obesity as a moral failing, lack of willpower, or character defect.

That's how it was supposed to work, in theory. But, strangely enough, obesity rates keep spiking. That's because the message hasn't gotten out, and healthcare providers don't view obesity as a disease. Yet, we know obesity is a disease because we can't always tie a person's excess fat to overeating and exercising too little.

Moreover, there isn't just one obesity type. Obesity subtypes include congenital, stress-induced, menopause-related, and MC4R-deficient, to name a few. See the box for definitions of each. But what they have in common is that they are all inflammatory states.

Obesity Sub-types

- Congenital obesity is more accurately described as congenital leptin deficiency, a rare genetic disorder in which someone can't produce leptin or produces it at very low levels. The absence of leptin signaling leads to an insatiable appetite and severe early-onset obesity.

- Stress-induced obesity is weight gain attributable to chronic stress. When the body experiences stress, it releases the hormone cortisol, which can increase appetite and cause the body to store fat, especially in the abdominal area. Research in the past ten years has shown stress to be associated with the presence of inflammatory mediators.

continued

- Menopause-related obesity refers to weight gain in women during and after menopause. During menopause, estrogen levels decline, which can lead to changes in body composition and metabolism, making weight gain easier and weight loss more challenging.

- MC4R-deficient obesity is a rare genetic obesity type affecting less than 1 percent of the population with obesity.[33] Mutations in the MC4R gene cause this type of obesity. Since MC4R-deficient obesity is a genetic disorder, it's incurable, but its symptoms can be managed with treatment.

Take-home Messages

Although BMI is often used to define obesity, as a disease obesity is not primarily a weight issue. Instead, obesity is a complex metabolic and behavioral disorder. It's always accompanied by inflammation, insulin resistance, and lipid abnormalities, including bad messaging between fat cells and the brain, ultimately leading to an increased risk of diabetes and cardiovascular disease.

So, while there is no quick and easy definition of obesity, I would like you to consider this: Obesity is a complex disease featuring an inflammatory state that compromises normal fat metabolism, hormone production, and responsiveness to important regulatory messages, leading to abnormal fat distribution, insulin resistance, and in most cases, increased weight. This complex disease is associated with various illnesses, including type 2 diabetes, atherosclerotic disease, and certain cancers.

Talley's Take: Should we call BS on BMI?

The scientific community has debated much about BMI and whether it's a valuable tool for assessing a person's health.

While it's a useful screening tool for population-level assessments and trends, BMI's application to individual health assessment has limitations. For example, BMI does not differentiate between lean body mass and fat mass. Therefore, two people with the same BMI may have different body compositions, and one may have a higher body fat percentage. BMI doesn't account for body fat distribution, age and gender differences, ethnic and population variations, and body composition changes over time. Other measures, such as cholesterol level, blood pressure, or insulin resistance, are far more accurate indicators of poor health and disease risk than BMI. Though BMI isn't a direct measure of health, higher BMI is generally associated with increased health risks, so it would be unwise to discount it entirely.

I work with many elite athletes. I gauge their fitness level by their body fat percentage, not their BMI. Many high-performance athletes who lift weights appear unhealthy based on their height-weight ratio. While I'm not a world-class athlete, I work out hard five or six days a week and carry a decent amount of muscle. At 6'2" and 235 pounds, my BMI is 30.17, placing me in the lower end of the obesity category. However, my body fat percentage is under 9 percent, an excellent score.

Body fat percentage (BFP) is the total mass of fat divided by total body mass. There are many ways to calculate BFP. First, you can try the waist-to-hip ratio. All you need is a tape measure and a simple calculation: *waist measurement divided by hip measurement*. We define high risk as a waist-hip ratio above 0.90 for men and above 0.85 for women. The downside of this measurement is that you have to calculate, and you need to know where to place the measuring tape:

measure the circumference of your hips at the widest point of your buttocks. For waist circumference, you must measure around the true waist, midway between the bottom of your ribs and the top of your hips.

You can also try a skinfold caliper, which measures the thickness of subcutaneous fat—the fat underneath the skin—at certain spots on the body. Calipers are the cheapest, easiest, and most portable method to measure body fat in specific areas. Skinfold measurements are generally taken on the right side of the body, with the tester pinching the skin at the location site. To try it, pick at least three spots on your body—chest, abs, and thigh are often used— pinch the skin, pull the fat away from the muscle, and measure the thickness of the fold with the calipers. I recommend taking an average of two measurements at each place. You then put those numbers into an online calculator, giving your body fat percentage.

In practice, using the skinfold measurements to monitor body fat over time is more beneficial than calculating your percent body fat each time. If your skinfold thickness drops, you are probably losing fat. The only downside of this measurement technique is that you have to be accurate, and humans aren't always so precise.

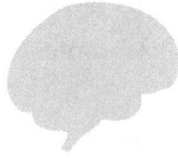

CHAPTER 3

Fat Map—Unraveling Obesity's Genetic Blueprint

"I'm not fat-shaming. I'm fat-splaining," said comedian and talk show host Bill Maher during a recent interview.

Maher, host of the popular HBO program *Real Time with Bill Maher*, has harshly critiqued the media's handling of America's weight problem, even accusing them of having "blood on their hands" for underreporting on obesity and COVID-19 death rates.

"Seventy-eight percent of the people who died or were hospitalized [with COVID] were obese," Maher said, adding that "the real epidemic is obesity, and that we don't talk about. We are at a different place with [obesity] than we were five years ago. Five years ago, it at least was thought to be a good thing to try to lose weight, right?

"Again, I'm not shaming people. I'm just saying we are never going to solve the healthcare crisis in this country until we get our arms around [obesity]."[1]

Responding to Maher's comments, actor and talk show host James Corden, who's spoken candidly about his weight struggles, delivered an almost eight-minute-long rant slamming the comedian's fat-shaming. Corden said he's never been able to control his weight despite his best efforts, confessing that he has "good days and bad months."[2]

So, which of them is correct? Are obese people to blame for their condition, as Maher seems to imply, or is something else happening?

Recent research suggests that obesity, or at least the propensity for extreme weight gain, is encoded in our genes, which dictate many of obesity's characteristic features. Indeed, identical twin studies show that obesity's heritability ranges between 70 and 80 percent, a level exceeded only by height.[3] The figure is higher than for many conditions we acknowledge as having a genetic basis, including sickle cell anemia and cystic fibrosis.

So, there it is. In some people, obesity, or at least the tendency to be obese, can be inherited. But as we will see, things are slightly more complicated than they might appear.

The Evidence

To date, scientists have uncovered over ninety new gene regions that could help explain why some people are more likely to put on weight than others.[4] That is a lot of places where something can go wrong. Obesity is seldom attributed to single-gene abnormalities; instead, there is a greater body of evidence suggesting that changes in multiple genes are at play.

In 2015, for example, scientists created a genetic "fat map" showing over sixty genetic locations influencing body mass index (BMI) alone.[5] A year later, University of California, San Francisco (UCSF), scientists took this information a step further, looking at the BMI-polygenic obesity risk relationship. First, researchers calculated a genetic risk score for each of the study subjects—7,482 white and 1,306 Black participants born between 1900 and 1958. The researchers determined the participants' risk scores using genetic variants linked to obesity and compared this with their BMI.

While BMI increased with age for everyone (until age sixty-five to sixty-nine), the average risk score did not change. However, within each age group, the BMI increase was greater for those with a higher risk score, and the overall pattern was similar regardless of race. Genes had a stronger effect on BMI for those born later.[6] These results tell me that genetic risk factors are only of limited importance in driving the obesity epidemic.

Genes play a role in BMI, and they also influence body fat distribution—a significant discovery given the connection to cardiovascular and metabolic diseases. Also, there are thirty-three gene regions linked to body fat distribution, explaining why some people are pear-shaped and others gain weight around the tummy.

In 2019, Uppsala University researchers in Sweden found that genetic factors play a significant role in determining fat storage, with a more pronounced impact observed in women. It is well recognized that fat distribution differs between genders, with women tending to store fat in the hips and legs, and men typically accumulating it around the abdomen, influenced by sex hormones like estrogen in women (while both men and women have androgenic hormones). Despite this knowledge, the precise molecular mechanisms governing these patterns remain relatively obscure.

In this study, researchers measured fat distribution in nearly 360,000 people. Participants gave blood samples for genotyping and researchers measured fat tissue distribution using electrical resistance. After examining millions of genetic variants, the researchers uncovered almost one hundred genes related to fat tissue distribution. Of note was the discovery of specific gene-encoded proteins that actively shape the extracellular matrix (the supporting material between the cells), suggesting that remodeling is one mechanism generating differences in body fat distribution.[7]

Perhaps the most persuasive argument for obesity's genetic antecedents comes from a British research team. They investigated the correlation between genomics and metabolite levels, which are molecules produced during the breakdown of food in the body. The team identified seventy-four genomic regions that were previously not known to influence the process of food breakdown into energy within our bodies.

The team used blood samples to measure 722 different metabolite levels—providing a snapshot of a person's well-being and the mechanisms that control critical physiological processes. For example, while nutrition, drugs, and the gut microbiome affect metabolite levels, a person's genes also affect how the body breaks down food.

This was not a small study. In fact, it was the largest-scale study of its kind looking at metabolism's genetic basis. From an independent 1,768-person cohort, researchers pinpointed more than 200 distinct genomic regions linked to variations in 478 different metabolite levels. Notably, some of these metabolites were found to be connected to BMI, offering additional understanding of the factors contributing to obesity. This breakthrough reveals fresh insights into the genetic influences on nutrient metabolism and offers valuable knowledge about how our bodies handle energy from the food we eat.[8]

Some researchers believe genetics outweigh environmental factors as we look at obesity's primary causes. They cite research showing that obesity between identical twins is consistent in up to 70 percent of cases. They believe that obesity-related genes have been identified since people with two copies of the so-called fat mass and obesity-associated (FTO) gene are heavier than those without the gene variant.[9] Moreover—and not surprisingly—sedentary people with the obesity-linked gene are heavier than those who are physically active.

So, why wouldn't researchers propose an obesity-related gene region? The evidence appears to be on their side. I can make an analogy with smoking to explain this point of view. If everyone inhaled the same amount of cigarette smoke every day, the most significant lung cancer risk factor would be a genetic susceptibility to the adverse effects of cigarette smoke.

However, this single gene theory cannot account for obesity's ever-increasing prevalence. For some, a genetic variant or mutation may be the root cause of their obesity, but that's not the case for most people.

Could a single gene variation be a cause of obesity?

For all the talk about multiple genes being a root cause of obesity, a recent National Institutes of Health (NIH) study points to a single and uncommon genetic variation as predisposing people to obesity.

NIH researchers found a variation of the appetite-regulating brain-derived neuropathic factor (BDNF) gene that produces lower levels of BDNF protein, which helps us feel full and may influence obesity in children and adults.

The researchers found an area of the gene where a single change reduced BDNF levels in the hypothalamus, a region of the brain that helps control eating and body weight.

Interestingly, the genetic change the researchers found wasn't a rare mutation but a variation occurring in the general

continued

population. Every living person has two copies, or alleles, of each gene they inherit from their parents. In their study, the researchers referred to the common allele as "T" and the less common allele, which produces less BDNF protein, as "C."

They compared a person's BDNF gene combination—CC, CT, or TT—to factors that define obesity, such as body mass index (BMI) and percentage of body fat.

The team found that the C allele was associated with higher BMI and body fat percentage in those with CT or CC types. In a group of healthy children of many races, the researchers found CC types had higher BMI scores and body fat percentages when compared with CT or TT types. Finally, the researchers found that the C allele (CT, CC types) was associated with higher BMI scores. Overall, the study suggests that the C allele of the BDNF gene may be linked to obesity.[10]

While this single variation may contribute to obesity in some people, the results don't point to the C allele as a root cause. What I gleaned from this study is that BDNF protein levels may offer a therapeutic strategy for people with the genetic variation, which occurs more often in African Americans and Hispanics than in Caucasians.

What about appetite control?

Could it be that thin people control their urge to eat, and obese people do not? If so, could this be genetically linked? Maybe, but the truth is far more complicated. Humans grow like weeds. Our body length increases by about 50 percent and our weight doubles during the first twelve months of life. Then the growth slows down until puberty. What drives this dynamic growth?

A recent study involving 30,000 Norwegian families reveals a link to the genes responsible for growth to extreme obesity, appetite, and energy intake.[11] The research could clarify why certain parents claim their children are hungrier than others and why they have more fat mass in infancy.

While genes may control early life appetite, these dynamic effects do not increase adult obesity risk. Once again, what looked so promising as proof of a simple, heritable genetic cause of obesity did not pan out.

These data show that a single gene doesn't predispose us to obesity, further explaining why one solution will not work for everyone.

Now, doctors use gender and age to make general recommendations about healthy living and weight. However, the data from this Norwegian study might allow us to give patients more tailored advice.

Can a hunger hormone imbalance cause obesity?

For anyone who doubts the Norwegian study's veracity or believes that being thin stems from greater self-control, consider the case of a four-year-old British boy who weighed 80 pounds, double the average weight for a boy his age, and his similarly affected 200-pound, eight-year-old cousin.

The two obese cousins' *hyperphasia*, or excessive eating, baffled doctors for years. Because of a very rare mutation in a crucial gene that produces leptin, a hormone that regulates fat storage and balances food intake and energy use, their hunger switch was always "on." However, after a few leptin injections, the four-year-old's calorie intake dropped to 180 per meal, and by the time he was six, his weight was in the normal range.

Nothing changed except for the boy's hormone levels. This boy was the victim of a faulty weight-regulating system that led to an uncontrollable drive to eat.[12]

The critical role of leptin in regulating eating behavior undermines the idea that food intake is under voluntary control.

Fat cells secrete leptin in normal-weight people, acting on specialized appetite-regulating brain cells. As fat percentage increases, there's a corresponding rise in leptin production and a drop in food intake. After weight loss, leptin levels drop, and appetite increases. Think of this physiologic system as a thermostat that maintains body weight within a relatively narrow range.

Mutations in these controlling genes rarely happen, and only a relative handful of patients don't produce leptin. However, mutations in brain tissue, where leptin exerts its effects, can also occur, including changes in the central nervous system's leptin receptor. For patients with these mutations, the receptors in their brains don't receive leptin's signal, and they subsequently become massively obese. Due to the impaired ability of these patients' brains to receive signals normally, hormone treatment proves ineffective. We characterize these patients as "leptin resistant." Again, this is very uncommon.

Changes in other key genes downstream of the hypothalamus can also cause human obesity. Recent studies have shown that up to 10 percent of markedly obese children carry mutations in one or another of these individual genes. So, when someone categorically asserts that "obesity isn't a birth defect" for these people, they're wrong.

The genes responsible for food intake and metabolism work together to keep a stable weight range by resisting weight change.

So, the more weight we lose, the hungrier we feel. During weight loss, the stomach releases greater amounts of the hormone called ghrelin, which makes us feel hungry. Ghrelin levels are higher in obese people, and these levels increase when these folks lose weight. If you think it's challenging to drop 15 pounds, imagine what it must feel like to lose 100 or 150—a situation confronting many obese patients.

Would a genetic test for obesity help?

There's a dream in medicine of diagnosing diseases—or at least predicting disease risk—with a simple DNA scan. But others say the practice, which could soon be a preventive medicine cornerstone, isn't worth the economic or emotional cost.

The thing to know about genetic obesity is single-gene mutations, such as activation of the MC4R gene, do not cause most inherited cases; instead, they derive from the cumulative effect of many genetic variants, an effect referred to as a polygenic inheritance. Genetic variants differ slightly from the same gene that determines specific traits, such as eye or hair color. Alone, each of those variants would have a relatively modest effect on weight, but together, their effects can have more dire consequences.

In 2019, researchers announced the creation of a tool—a genome-wide polygenic score (GPS)—that forecasts a person's genetic susceptibility to weight gain from early life into adulthood. This predictive tool could offer new opportunities to improve clinical prevention and provide insights into genetic obesity's underlying causes.[13]

Although the basic facts are not in dispute—our genes play a crucial role in extreme weight gain—the problem with obesity is that, unlike diseases caused by a single gene gone haywire, thousands of genes increase obesity risk. Conversely, single gene variants contribute only a minuscule risk. So, is it worth diving deep into DNA databanks when there's no obvious way to put that information to good use?

A recent study of over 300,000 people by Harvard and Broad Institute researchers found over 2 million DNA variants of potential interest. While most are irrelevant, researchers suspect small mutations are hiding somewhere in this vast genetic haystack that, together or individually, contributes to a person's obesity risk.

Since thousands of genes play a role in obesity, no single gene can do much to move the needle. But taken together, the information gathered could be potentially helpful. For example, in the Harvard study, folks with the highest risk scores (those with the most variants) were more likely to be severely obese (with a BMI over 40). In fact, 43 percent of the study participants with the highest genetic risk scores were obese. However, the test had its downsides. For instance, 17 percent of the subjects with the highest scores had normal body weights.

Early childhood is a crucial time to begin obesity prevention efforts, as genetics play a role during this stage, say the researchers. However, I think early childhood is much too late to begin obesity prevention efforts. A recent meta-analysis concluded that without a greater emphasis on prevention, 57 percent of today's children will be obese by age thirty-five.[14, 15]

Another View

While the Harvard study was the first of its kind, scientists already knew genetic risk factors could contribute significantly to obesity. However, I think little of the strategy of coming up with a cumulative risk score by adding up the miniscule risks millions of genetic variants pose. My skepticism comes from the fact that no one knows if all these variants matter. Obesity is a multifactorial illness, and putting too much emphasis on a single cause (such as genetics) might prove more of a hindrance than a help.

Also, the Harvard study revealed nothing about the individual genes contributing to obesity, so you can't use the results to understand the disease's underlying biology. If obesity were a rare disease, such as Tay-Sachs, a test could help identify people at elevated risk. But since obesity reportedly affects at least 43 percent of Americans (I suspect the actual number is higher), prevention efforts should be all-encompassing.

Showing a solid statistical correlation is one thing. Using that information to change behavior positively is another matter entirely. Experience has taught me that personalized risk information has a negligible effect on human behavior. It all boils down to how we perceive and process risk. Humans often exhibit cognitive biases that can affect their risk perception, such as optimism bias or the tendency to believe that adverse events are less likely to happen to them.

Moreover, we have different thresholds for what we consider a significant risk. Some may downplay or ignore risks that do not align with their pre-existing beliefs or preferences. Additionally, the presentation of risk information, including the format and framing, can influence its impact. If the data are too complex or presented in a problematic way, people may struggle to incorporate it into their decision-making process.

Behavioral factors such as emotions, social influences, and immediate rewards also play a crucial role. Personalized risk information might not effectively address these factors or may be overshadowed by more immediate concerns and motivations.

A Final Word

While there's a clear genetic link to obesity, we still don't know the specific genes that contribute to extreme weight gain. It is clear from all the research that there is no "fat gene." Many different genes are involved, and in the next chapter we will see how this happens.

Just as attitudes toward depression have changed in recent years, we're now on the way to viewing obesity as a disease, not a personal shortcoming. For this reason alone, I believe that this genetic theory of obesity has made us smarter about obesity's root causes. As I will show you in the next chapter, an altered or mutated gene is seldom the guilty party.

Talley's Take: Is it really all in the genes?

"They said I need to lose weight."

My client, a leading NBA player with a history of injury problems, was told by team physicians and trainers that his inability to stay on the court starts and ends with the extra 30 pounds he's carrying on his 6'6" frame.

This player's weight is so problematic that his team added a clause to his recent contract extension. He must keep his body weight and body fat percentage at a certain level—the team insists on regular weigh-ins—or else they would reduce his guaranteed salary. Another client, one of the world's leading boxers, was so concerned about his weight that he didn't want to fight shirtless.

When my NBA client came to my office, he expressed frustration with the team's insistence on a weight clause.

"I'm trying to keep my weight down, but it's hard. I was born this way. Everybody in my immediate family has a weight problem. So, what am I supposed to do?" he said.

I told him while it's true that several people in his family struggle with weight problems, it's unlikely that genetics is the culprit. And that is good news, because that meant it would be easier to do something about the challenges facing him.

"We can't change your genes, but we can change their expression, including those that might predispose you to weight gain. So just changing your environment and behaviors, such as eating a healthier diet and doing more off-court physical training, will help. Also, giving you strategies to break some of the negative habits you've gotten into, like eating out of boredom and mindless snacking, can cause epigenetic changes that might make it easier for you to lose weight and keep it off."

We've been working together for eighteen months, and I'm happy to report my client is down 35 pounds and has no sign of slipping back into the old habits and behaviors that got him into trouble.

Here are my two cents on obesity's genetic contributions: A heightened understanding of obesity's genetics and gene-environment interactions will give us a better understanding of the disease's causal pathways, of which there are many. Such information could help us develop better obesity prevention and treatment modalities. However, we should acknowledge that our genes' contribution to obesity risk is minimal, while many other variables, including transgenerational epigenetic inheritance and an increasingly toxic environment, are significant. Genes may co-determine who becomes obese, but our environment determines how many become obese.

I told my client, as I tell everyone, to stop worrying about the imaginary albatross around his neck or thinking that he's resigned to a lifetime of weight problems. Our genes aren't our destiny. We have the power to change course and enjoy a healthier future.

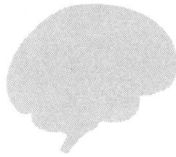

CHAPTER 4

You Are What Your Mother Ate— The Role of Epigenetics on Obesity

H ave you ever wondered why you are the way you are? No, I'm not talking about eye color, hair color, or height. Instead, I'm thinking about other things. Why are you calm or anxious? Why are you energetic? Why are you always lethargic? Why are you thin? Why do you struggle to lose weight?

There are many answers to these questions. We are the way we are because of our genes—the DNA we inherited at conception. However, we turn out the way we do because of our experiences— how others treated us and what entered our bodies, especially during those crucial first years of life . . . even as a fetus.

I make the point in the previous chapter that obesity is heritable and often runs in families. At least a dozen genetic variants increase a person's risk of being overweight or obese. However, I suggest you pause if you think your DNA is solely responsible for your weight problems. Indeed, it's rarely the case that obesity can be chalked up entirely to bad genes. Research shows that genetic variants only account for a small percentage of inherited obesity. So, if 40 to 70 percent of people carry the so-called "obesity genes," a sizable part of heritability remains unexplained.[1] Are children similar to their parents because they share the same lifestyles? Or is something else at play?

Heredity might influence whether our bodies become obese or lean, but the genes that researchers link to extra pounds don't explain weight differences among people. For example, identical twins, alike in everything from their eye color to their favorite foods and even their predisposition to substance abuse, can diverge in one important characteristic: their weight.[2]

What accounts for the variation? To fully understand how obesity develops, we must look beyond the simple DNA sequence we all inherit.

What is epigenetics?

DNA is the human body's instruction manual. However, genes need help to know what to do, and where and when to do it. For example, a human liver cell contains the same DNA as a lung cell, yet somehow it knows to code only those proteins needed for the liver's functioning. You won't find those instructions in our DNA. Instead, they're found on the DNA in a complex array of chemical markers and switches, which collectively make up the epigenome. The epigenome is a hodgepodge of chemical compounds that modify, or mark, the genome in a way that tells it what to do, where to do it, and when to do it.[3]

Think of the epigenome as a complex software code that instructs the DNA hardware to manufacture an impressive variety of proteins, cell types, and individuals. The even greater surprise is the recent discovery that epigenetic signals can be passed on from one generation to the next, sometimes for several generations, without changing a single gene sequence. For example, we know that environmental effects, such as radiation, alter the expression of the genetic sequences in a sex cell's DNA and can leave a mark on future generations.[4]

Likewise, the intrauterine environment impacts a fetus's development. What's eye-opening—and what several animal studies show—is evidence suggesting that the epigenetic changes spurred by diet, behavior, or surroundings can work their way into the germ line and reverberate far into the future. And as bizarre as it may sound, what you eat, drink, smoke, or expose yourself to today could affect your great-grandchildren's health and behavior.

In recent years, science has made remarkable progress toward understanding the molecular sequences and patterns that determine gene activation or deactivation. This work has clarified that for all the widespread attention devoted to genome-sequencing projects, the epigenome is just as critical as DNA to an organism's healthy development. And by "organism," I mean humans as well.

So, you might wonder, what role does epigenetics play in human obesity? Well, I'm glad you asked. We can pass down environmentally triggered epigenetic modifications from one generation to the next. This transmission type happened in China during the Great Chinese Famine of 1959–1961, when somewhere between 15 and 45 million people (about twice the population of New York State) died of hunger from a number of causes during the era of Mao Zedong. Many children born during this time were small and underweight, most likely because of poor in-utero nutrition. However, they also had a significantly increased risk of hyperglycemia and type 2 diabetes, conditions characteristic of obesity.[5]

So, what happened here? Research suggests that while in utero, epigenetic factors might have altered IGF2DMR, a gene that controls appetite, metabolism, and digestion. These children now had a built-in mechanism to prepare for the next famine, upregulating the genes for storing energy as fat, just in case.

It's worth mentioning that the increased methylation (the attachment of methyl groups) on the IGF2DMR gene occurred during the first trimester following exposure to a severe famine, suggesting that epigenetic marks may be most influential during early gestation, when the genome is more vulnerable. Developing tissue is fertile ground for these epigenetic changes.[6]

Bottom line: mothers pregnant during the famine gave birth to children who, decades later, are especially obesity-prone, suggesting that the mothers' diets had a lasting impact on their offspring's metabolism.

I've long suspected that epigenetics was a root cause of the global obesity epidemic, and here's why. For years, the ratio of obese to lean people in our obesogenic environment has remained stable, suggesting individual variation and predisposition. Epigenome-wide association studies (EWAS) have identified more epigenetic than genetic obesity-associated changes.[7] Several animal studies and even a few involving humans demonstrate epigenetic modification effects, including DNA methylation, have a profound effect on obesity. Let's look at those so you can understand my predisposition.

Animal Models and Epigenetics

Animal models are helpful because they allow us to gather data that would be impossible to extract from humans. We also use animal models because humans and animals share much of their DNA, underscoring our kinship. We're so similar that we share about 70 percent of our genes with two acorn worm species.

Evidence suggests that mammals cloned for clinical studies are typically heavier with adult-onset obesity. However, nothing has changed in these animals' DNA sequencing. Instead, outside factors have affected their genes' expression.

In 2000, Randy Jirtle, a Duke University professor, designed a groundbreaking genetic experiment that was simplicity personified. Dr. Jirtle used pairs of fat yellow mice known to scientists as agouti mice because they carry a particular gene—the agouti gene—that leaves them prone to cancer and diabetes while making the rodents ravenous and yellow.

Dr. Jirtle wanted to see if he could reshape these little critters' unfortunate genetic legacy. Usually, when agouti mice breed, the offspring are identical to the parents—yellow, fat, and susceptible to life-shortening diseases. However, these parents also produced some offspring that looked different. These young mice were slender and brown. But, more significantly, they did not display their parents' susceptibility to cancer and diabetes and lived to a spry old mouse age.

What does this mean? It means a virtual erasure of the agouti gene's effects. Remarkably, the researchers elicited this transformation without altering a single letter of the mouse's DNA! Their approach instead was radically straightforward—they changed the mother mouse's diet. Starting just before conception, Dr. Jirtle fed a test group of mother mice a diet rich in methyl donors, the small chemical clusters that attach to a gene and can turn it on or off. Many foods, including onions, garlic, and beets, contain these donors, as do food supplements such as folic acid, which we give to pregnant women. After being consumed by the mother mice, the methyl donors worked their way into the developing embryos' chromosomes and onto the surface of the critical agouti gene. The mothers passed along the agouti gene to their offspring, but thanks to their methyl-rich pregnancy diet, they had added a chemical switch to the gene that dimmed its harmful effects. It's hard to believe that something as seemingly innocuous as a nutritional change in a pregnant mouse could dramatically affect her offspring's gene expression. These results showed how powerful epigenetic changes can be.[8, 9]

Dr. Jirtle's study and others like it looking into epigenetics' influence on weight show multiple gestational exposures that could induce changes that persist after birth. So, decades later, an odd pattern of weight gain in some mutant mice intrigued researchers at the famed Max Planck Institute of Immunobiology and Epigenetics in Freiburg, Germany. The mice had only one copy of a gene called Trim28, and the researchers found that most of them were either obese or lean, with a few animals in the midrange. Some genes' job is to control other genes' activity. Trim28 does that. It's an epigenetic modifier. Researchers at the Planck Institute found that Trim28 turns down the activity of an interacting set of genes in obese mice. Earlier studies tied these genes to body weight management, and some are activated in fat cells and the hypothalamus, the brain area that controls hunger. The genes' function is still unclear, but the German researchers speculate that Trim28 helps form an epigenetic switch that can flip on obesity by suppressing these genes.

But could the identical epigenetic mechanism contribute to human obesity? It seems like a reasonable conclusion. After all, mice have only one copy of the Trim28 gene, while people have two copies. The Max Planck research team took fat samples from pediatric surgical patients and observed abnormally low Trim28 activity in obese children's fat.

The researchers also analyzed data on thirteen pairs of identical twins in which one was obese. Trim28 activity was less in the obese twins' fat, the researchers reported.[10]

All this research shows that you can have a strong phenotype (in this case, obesity) with no genetic underpinnings. Scientists once thought epigenetic effects might tweak our weight by only a few pounds. However, if people packed on pounds equivalent to what the mice gained, it would mean the difference between a heavyweight boxer versus a welterweight. These studies and others like them introduced a new potential mechanism for obesity's development.

Making Sense

Dr. Jirtle's experiment was a benchmark demonstration that the epigenome is sensitive to environmental cues. Increasingly, researchers find that an extra bit of a vitamin, a brief exposure to a chemical toxin, or even an added dose of mothering can tweak the epigenome—and alter our genes' software—in ways that affect an individual's body and brain for life. These discoveries are shaking the modern biological and social understandings about genetics and identity. We commonly accept that DNA is a life sentence, predisposing us to certain body shapes, personalities, and diseases. Some scholars even contend that the genetic code predetermines intelligence and is the root cause of many social ills, including poverty, crime, and violence.

While "genes as destiny" is still conventional medical wisdom in some circles, thanks to what we now know about epigenetics, that notion is outdated. Epigenetics proves we have some influence over our genome's integrity and expression, which is good news for the millions who are obese. Before, we thought genes predetermined outcomes. Now we know that everything we do and everything we're exposed to can affect our gene expression and those of future generations. Epigenetics introduces the concept of free will into the genetics conversation.

Scientists still don't fully understand how epigenetic changes unfold at the biochemical level, but they are learning. For example, one form of epigenetic modification physically blocks access to the genes by altering the histone code. The DNA in every cell is tightly wound around proteins known as histones, and this histone wrapping must be unwound before the enzyme RNA polymerase can transcribe them. Alterations to this packaging cause specific genes to be more or less available to methyl groups or other epigenetic factors.

The best-understood form of epigenetic signaling, DNA methylation, involves adding a methyl group—a carbon atom plus three hydrogen atoms—to respective bases in the DNA sequence. Methylation interferes with the chemical signals that put the gene into action, effectively silencing it.

Epigenetics explains how little things can have an effect of great magnitude. Indeed, epigenetic patterns can shift throughout life, and those changes are an important part of the development and dissemination of diseases such as diabetes, cancer, and obesity. Tumors, for example, metastasize following the methylation of tumor-suppressing genes.

Likewise, the demethylation of genes that typically promote tumor growth—which removes the dimmer switches usually present—kicks those genes into action, causing tumor growth. It's no accident that we find abnormal methylation patterns in many colon, stomach, cervix, prostate, thyroid, and breast cancers.[11]

DNA Methylation's Role in the Obesity Epidemic

DNA methylation is the epigenetic mechanism that most profoundly affects obesity. In 2019, an international research team compared obese and lean mice and found differing methylation patterns in several hundred regions. When the researchers compared fat cells from obese and lean humans, they found the same pattern.

The same researchers found that many epigenetic changes that promote obesity also raise diabetes risk. They compared before and after samples from obese gastric bypass patients and found that many of the obese-type methylation patterns reverted to lean-type patterns post-surgery. The surgery appears to have altered the epigenome.

In a separate study, researchers compared the methylation patterns in pancreatic islets of healthy individuals and patients with type 2 diabetes. The analysis revealed epigenetic changes in about eight hundred genes in people with type 2 diabetes. Over one hundred of these genes had altered expression, many of them in ways that could contribute to reduced insulin production.[12]

In another study, researchers looked at the methylation patterns of fourteen pairs of identical adult twins, one healthy and one with type 2 diabetes. Although the twins had similar methylation patterns, the diabetic siblings showed upregulation of the genes involved in inflammation, and downregulation of those involved in fat and glucose metabolism. The researchers believe that lifestyle choices account for the differences.[13]

The Real Value of Exercise

In a first-of-its-kind study, scientists examined how exercise changes methyl groups in fat cells. The study involved twenty-three slightly overweight but otherwise healthy men in their mid-thirties who had low levels of physical activity. For six months, the men attended aerobic exercise classes an average of twice a week and showed improved fitness and weight loss without dietary changes.

Looking at the men's before and after cell samples, the researchers found changes in 7,000 genes' methylation patterns, including beneficial alterations in many genes linked to diabetes and obesity. The researchers confirmed the findings using lab studies of other fat cells, in which they silenced some implicated genes, resulting in changes in insulin sensitivity and fat storage.[14] This study shows exercise's value for people who are obese or overweight. Exercise changes the epigenetic pattern of genes affecting fat storage.

Obesity Heritability

By now, it should be obvious that epigenetic changes are heritable. But don't think about this as a question of nature versus nurture. Instead, the parents' obesity—independent of their DNA—affects a child's epigenome.

Maternal glucose levels, maternal weight gain, environmental exposures, and too little or too much food intake before and during pregnancy can increase childhood obesity in offspring. Studies have also shown that the methylation pattern of specific genes in cord blood samples of newborns correlates with childhood obesity.[15] Many factors may affect how genes are expressed or silenced, secondary to factors during pregnancy. I am telling you that things you do before conceiving a child could also influence that child's obesity risk.

Let's look at dads for a moment. Most people view the dad's role in conception as little more than sperm donation. They don't consider the father's health contributing to the child's future health. Moms unfairly shoulder much of this burden. However, we can't overstate the sperm's role in childhood development. Indeed, many studies show that a man's health can significantly affect his children's and grandchildren's health.

One commonly cited study followed a series of Swedish citizens born in 1890, 1905, and 1920, respectively. The researchers tracked the kids of this study group and then studied their kids until 1995. The study aimed to assess if food intake during a father's prepubescent slow growth period affected his child and grandchild's obesity risk. It turns out it did. Those dads exposed to a limited amount of food during their slow growth period had kids with a reduced risk of cardiovascular disease. But those with too much food during the same period had grandkids with increased type 2 diabetes risk.

More recent mouse studies further show paternal nutrition's influence on future generations' health. In these studies, male mice fed high-fat, low-protein diets sired offspring with a higher fatty liver composition. They also showed that paternal mice fed obesity-inducing diets had grandchildren with more fat at birth.[16]

A study by Danish researchers published in the journal *Cell Metabolism* implicates an epigenetic mechanism in sperm that might influence childhood obesity's development. A comparison of the sperm of thirteen normal-weight and ten obese kids showed a "distinct epigenome that characterizes human obesity." Small non-coding RNA characterized this epigenome.[17]

The study also looked at the sperm of morbidly obese men who underwent gastric bypass, both before the surgery and again a year later, after weight loss. Again, they found "a dramatic remodeling of sperm DNA methylation, notably at genetic locations implicated in the central control of appetite" toward the lean type.[18]

These data suggest that the parents' pre-conception lifestyle and dietary habits profoundly influence obesity's development in their children and grandchildren. Interestingly, the researchers' data also show that developing sperm may be susceptible to environmental insults. These findings are of considerable importance because these changes may be passed on to the next generation, increasing the risk for chronic diseases such as obesity.[19]

The data from these studies also suggest that methylation levels in the gene involved in lipid metabolism—lipoprotein lipase (LPL)—are higher in obese people with type 2 diabetes. Since LPL determines whether our tissues store or consume ingested fat, dysfunction of this gene would cause high blood triglyceride levels.

This study also shows lower DNA methylation in genes related to inflammatory processes, such as tumor necrosis factor (TNF). Low methylation may cause a higher functioning of this gene, which may affect the pro-inflammatory condition observed in obese people who also have an associated metabolic disease.

These are exciting findings. However, we can't forget that correlation doesn't equal causation. Teasing out causes will take more time and effort.

What You Can Do—The Importance of Epigenetic Regulation

Many of you may read these words and think that all is lost, and no amount of diet and exercise could help reverse these epigenetic changes. Right? Fortunately, that's not the case. Of course, we can't change how our grandparents ate, exercised, or their environmental exposures, which may affect our genes' expression. However, we can influence our current dietary and exercise habits and limit our toxic exposures to help future generations. The good news is that, unlike genetic mutations, epigenetic changes are reversible.

Both nutrition and exercise are critical environmental factors that can positively and negatively affect our gene expression at every stage of development. Some researchers are looking into so-called "methylation diets" to help prevent extreme weight gain. We could tailor such a diet to a person's genetic makeup and exposure to environmental toxins. Even something as simple as adding one food could make a difference. For example, a Rutgers University study looked at the epigenetic effects of green tea—the first study to demonstrate that a consumer product could inhibit DNA methylation.[20] Genistein, resveratrol, curcumin, and other compounds in many popular foods show similar epigenetic effects.

Practical Steps

So, what can you do? Knowing that maternal weight gain during pregnancy and glucose control affect childhood obesity risk, a mom can still manage her eating and exercise habits during pregnancy to improve these outcomes. Normal weight gain after the first trimester is about a pound per week. Too much weight gain in the first trimester can have adverse effects. Gestational diabetes during pregnancy doesn't automatically lead to negative epigenetic factors for the unborn infant, but it's something to avoid if possible. Healthy eating, exercise, and possibly medications can improve the developing fetus's glucose and leptin levels.

For dads, it's not that difficult. Be healthy. Seriously. Take care of your diet. Get regular exercise. Limit drug and alcohol use. Or, better yet, abstain altogether. You never know when you might conceive a child, and since our sperm turns over constantly, it's essential to have the least negative epigenetic factors present when it happens.

Other things that might help include the development of epigenetic drugs. One such drug, 5-azacytidine, has been approved for myelodysplastic syndrome, also known as preleukemia or smoldering leukemia. At least eight other epigenetic drugs are currently in different stages of development or human trials. Methylation patterns also hold promise as diagnostic tools, potentially yielding critical information about the odds that obesity will respond to treatment.

Another exciting idea is the Human Epigenome Project, which would map our entire epigenome. However, this would be a massive undertaking. The Human Genome Project, which sequenced the 3 billion pairs of nucleotide bases in human DNA, was a piece of cake by comparison. Epigenetic markers and patterns are different in every tissue type in the human body, not to mention they change. We don't have one epigenome; we have a multitude of them.

I still consider epigenetics a young field. There is a lot of information we still don't understand. We are still learning how to manipulate the epigenome to get the positive results we want. We know that the healthier we are as parents, the healthier our kids will be. Early on, teach your children the value of healthy eating. Keep them active. The information above is just a tiny amount of the data available involving epigenetics and the human genome. Factors like toxic stress, environmental exposures, placental changes, and other influences can positively or negatively affect our genomic expression.

A Final Thought

Understanding and possibly manipulating our epigenetics presents us with the best opportunity to do something about the obesity epidemic. It's time to abandon the idea that DNA is the only form of information we inherit from our parents. We inherit far more than DNA—we inherit chromosomes, which are only 50 percent of DNA. The other 50 percent are protein molecules, and these proteins also carry epigenetic marks and information. So, the entire chromosome is an open target for epigenetic changes, and the chromosome is what we pass on to future generations.

Talley's Take: Navigating the Epigenetic Exercise Landscape

As you know from reading this chapter, epigenetic changes always happen. Diet, obesity, physical activity, tobacco smoking, alcohol consumption, environmental pollutants, psychological stress, and night shift work influence epigenetic patterns. However, they're a normal response to a person's ambient environment. For instance, a person living in Steamboat Springs, Colorado, which sits 6,732 feet (about 2.05 km) above sea level, will have more red blood cells in his bloodstream because the low oxygen levels affect his genes' expression. We see similar epigenetic changes in professional mountain climbers.

However, you don't have to be a professional mountain climber to reap exercise's epigenetic benefits. I routinely see gene expression changes in high-performance athletes and ordinary people who make tangible, lasting lifestyle changes.

Indeed, two of my clients—professional soccer player Ellen, and weekend warrior Curtis (who runs, cycles, and plays a mean game of tennis)—use targeted exercises to improve their health. Both athletes are on a resistance training program that includes squats, lunges, chin-ups, push-ups, and planks. These exercises induce epigenetic changes that improve energy metabolism, muscle development, and insulin sensitivity, contributing to healthy skeletal muscle. For mixed endurance sports such as soccer and tennis, fartlek training—a kind of running training which involves random variations in speed and intensity, alternating between bursts of sprinting and slower "recovery" jogging or walking—is also helpful.

Since Curtis is carrying a few extra pounds—his BMI sometimes flirts in the lower obese range—the resistance exercises help with excess fat loss by increasing both after-burn and muscle size.

As a professional athlete, Ellen's needs and training habits are different—she exercises for a living—but the training offers her the same benefits.

The other good news about exercise is that it works in the short and long term to prevent metabolic diseases such as obesity and improve overall health. However, the most substantial epigenetic benefits come from a lifetime commitment to regular exercise. For example, running and cycling over a long period of time can change the activity of more than 1,000 genes.

However, even a short exercise program is enough to alter a person's skeletal muscle profile to a point where it more closely resembles those of long-term endurance trainers. For obese and overweight people, short exercise programs can positively influence their metabolic profiles, improving their overall health.

I tell my clients that consistency is key here. That's why anyone looking to start an exercise regimen should choose something they'll stick with. To succeed, pick an activity you would do as routinely as eating, sleeping, brushing your teeth, or showering. Also, you don't need a daily two-hour-long sweat session to see positive changes. For example, walking, meditation, tai chi, and yoga produce wide-ranging gene expression changes, such as slowing age-related gene methylation.

CHAPTER 5

Waist Dump—Environmental Toxins' Impact on the Obesity Epidemic

What if I told you that the most dangerous thing for your weight—and what might put you at the greatest risk for obesity—has nothing to do with what you put in your mouth? Better yet, would you believe that dozens of consumer products, many of which are in your home right now, contribute to obesity? Could something as benign as drink bottles, yogurt tubs, and freezer bags be contributing to the global obesity epidemic? It's not only possible; mounting evidence suggests it's true.

Until recently, such a notion would have seemed absurd. But a mounting body of evidence suggests that chemical exposures that disrupt the function of some hormones, particularly during prenatal development, may be a predisposing factor for weight gain and related metabolic health problems.

These endocrine-disrupting chemicals (EDCs), commonly referred to as obesogens, are indeed ubiquitous and found widely throughout our environment. EDCs mimic, block, or alter the action of natural hormones, leading to disruptions in various physiological processes.

They're abundant in water and dust, household cleaners, furniture, and electronics. They also lurk in pesticides, flame retardants, antifouling paints, plastic compounds, and detergents. A recent study found that eleven substances in everyday products, including sponges and trashcan liners, can reprogram stem cells in a developing fetus to become fat cells, which then multiply, introducing more fat.[1] Imagine that!

Obesogens influence weight gain and metabolic health via several mechanisms. They can interfere with the endocrine system, affecting the production, release, and function of hormones that play a role in metabolism, appetite, and fat storage. Obesogen exposure during critical early life periods such as prenatal or early postnatal development can lead to epigenetic modifications, altering gene expression related to metabolic processes. Obesogens may promote the formation of new fat cells (adipogenesis) and increase the size of existing fat cells, contributing to weight gain and obesity. Some obesogens can affect the central nervous system, also influencing appetite and overeating. Obesogens have been linked to insulin resistance, a complex condition in which the body's cells become less responsive to insulin, triggering elevated blood sugar levels and an increased risk of type 2 diabetes.

Common obesogens such as phthalates, which are found in personal care products, electronics, and food packaging, can reprogram how our bodies metabolize protein, pushing our bodies to store fat, regardless of physical activity level or diet. Perfluorooctane sulfonic acid (PFOS), present in non-stick cookware, water-resistant clothing, and furniture coatings designed to repel spills, deceives our bodies into retaining fat, even when external circumstances suggest that we should be burning calories. In adults who lost weight following a healthy diet with physical activity, higher PFOS concentrations at baseline increased the likelihood of weight regain over a two-year follow-up period, according to a 2018 study.[2]

And this list only scratches the surface.

Fat Factors: How Obesogens Work

As you read this chapter, you might wonder how plastic containers or cosmetics can cause weight gain.

In 2005, a research team at Washington State University, led by microbiologist Michael Skinner, made a groundbreaking discovery in the field of obesogen science. Their research uncovered that pregnant rats exposed to increased concentrations of the widely used fungicide vinclozolin produced male offspring with consistently reduced sperm counts in successive generations. Furthermore, they noticed changes in DNA methylation patterns in the reproductive cell line. Intrigued by the effects of various environmental chemicals, they conducted screenings that included toxic substances like jet fuel, plastic additives, and additional pesticides, discovering that exposed animals continued to pass down reproductive problems and frequently exhibited obesity as another recurring phenotype.[3]

This experiment wasn't Dr. Skinner's only fat rat encounter. He first saw the corpulent critters in his experiments after injecting female rats with bisphenol A and phthalates. The rats' kids and their grandkids—animals not directly exposed to the chemicals—showed other abnormalities but were of normal weight. However, roughly 10 percent of the grandkid rats descended from exposed females became obese.[4]

The research team also tested DDT, a once widely used pesticide banned in the US in the 1970s because of its impact on bird populations and concerns that it could harm human health. Rats whose mothers or grandmothers were exposed to the chemical had normal body sizes. However, just a generation later, 50 percent of the population was obese.

What Dr. Skinner's findings affirmed is that altered inheritance does not occur the way many of us were taught. Instead of changing the DNA sequences that make up the genes that ancestors pass down to descendants, something more subtle occurs: transgenerational epigenetic inheritance! A life experience—in Dr. Skinner's study, exposing rats to vinclozolin—alters the on-off switches that control sperm and egg DNA.

Biologists have long known about epigenetic switches, which are controlled by atom clusters called methyl groups. The cluster can silence a gene it attaches to; when the cluster is removed, the gene becomes active again. (This silencing is why the DNA for, say, insulin can be turned off in brain cells but active in pancreas cells.) For many years biologists believed that when sperm and eggs matured, as it were, and created an embryo, the methyl group tags were reset—nature's way of erasing the sins of the fathers and mothers before they could afflict the next generation. They believed that genes were effectively "stripped" of their epigenetic tags.

Dr. Skinner's discovery proved otherwise—that all those marks aren't erased but are instead indefinitely modified (they continued through four rat generations)—and challenged a bedrock tenant of reproductive biology. Along the way, Dr. Skinner became the forerunner of a new way of thinking about the possible long-term health consequences of environmental chemical exposures.

Dr. Skinner's findings weren't anomalous. Dr. Robert Sargis, an associate professor at the University of Illinois College of Medicine, explored the effects of environmental endocrine disruptors, specifically obesogens, on glucocorticoid signaling pathways, which are involved in fat-cell differentiation and lipid accumulation.

Dr. Sargis's research focused on four specific compounds:

1. **BPA (Bisphenol A):** BPA is a chemical used in the production of plastics and resins. It has been known to act as an endocrine disruptor, mimicking estrogen and affecting hormone pathways in the body.

2. **Dicyclohexyl phthalate:** This is a plasticizer, a type of chemical commonly used to make plastics more flexible. Like BPA, phthalates are also known endocrine disruptors.

3. **Endrin:** Endrin is an organochlorine pesticide that was once widely used in agriculture. It has been banned in several countries due to its toxic effects on the environment and potential health risks.

4. **Tolylfluanid:** Tolylfluanid is a fungicide used in agriculture to protect crops from fungal diseases. It is also an endocrine disruptor.

Dr. Sargis discovered that each of these four compounds activated the glucocorticoid receptor, which is involved in regulating various metabolic processes, including fat-cell differentiation and lipid accumulation. When these compounds activate the glucocorticoid receptor it can disrupt the body's hormonal balance, potentially contributing to obesity and metabolic problems.[5]

Of Mice and Obesogens

Determining obesogens' exact contribution to the obesity epidemic is challenging, but several scientists have a good idea. The word "obesogen" first emerged in 2006 when Bruce Blumberg, PhD, professor of developmental and cell biology at the University of California, Irvine, made a disturbing discovery in his laboratory.

Tin-based compounds, known as organotins, were significantly impacting the weight of laboratory mice. This influence was so potent that mice exposed to these organotins while in the womb, even when fed a regular diet, ended up weighing approximately 15 percent more than the unexposed mice. Fifteen percent might not seem like much, but as Dr. Blumberg pointed out, it's the difference between what we weighed a generation ago and where we are now.

In 2006, Dr. Blumberg and his colleague Felix Grün applied the term obesogen to a variety of chemicals, including tributyltin (TBT), a fungicide used to prevent barnacle encrustation on boat hulls, docks, and fishing nets. TBT was also used for slime control in paper mills, disinfection of circulating industrial cooling waters, and wood preservation. The two researchers found that feeding pregnant mice just a single dose produced offspring born with greater fat stores than normal. At ten weeks of age, these mice weighed about 15 percent more than unexposed mice.[6]

Equally if not more worrisome was the trend Dr. Blumberg and his colleagues discovered when they followed these prenatally exposed mice through subsequent generations. The mice born to the second generation of heavier mice (that is, the mice who had been exposed to TBT in utero) were also fatter—even though they'd had zero direct prenatal TBT exposure. Even back in 2006, the reason for this phenomenon was obvious to Dr. Blumberg and his colleagues. When you expose a pregnant female, you also expose her fetus's immature sex cells (germ cells), which will one day be her grandchildren. These epigenetically altered egg cells gave rise to a third generation of fatter mice. And here's one more thing Dr. Blumberg unearthed. When the fatter third-generation mice had babies, they were also fatter—even though this fourth generation had no direct chemical exposure, not even indirectly through their mothers. Dr. Blumberg said, and I believe he's spot-on, that once this epigenetic change makes its way to the great-grandchildren, it's effectively permanent.

When the Math Doesn't Add Up

You rarely find consensus amongst scientists. But nearly all I speak with agree that obesity is a problem. However, that's where the consensus breaks down. There's much debate about why obesity has reached epidemic proportions. If it's true that the availability of calorie-rich, mass-produced, and highly palatable foods is the root cause of obesity, then I'd like to know how these foods contribute to excess body fat for one simple reason: over the past twenty years, calorie intake by US adults has remained constant (even trending slightly down).[7]

How do we explain this disparity? The problem with the energy balance model is that it's a house of cards—just the slightest scrutiny and everything comes tumbling down. If the energy balance model were accurate, we should expect declining obesity rates since we're not eating more today than we were twenty years ago when 32.2 percent of US adults (about 66.5 million) were obese.[8] But obesity rates are skyrocketing and expected to climb to 51 percent both at home and abroad, or over 4 billion people, within the next twelve years.[9] So, I return to my earlier question: Why do we keep gaining weight?

In our pursuit of understanding and addressing the escalating obesity epidemic, it is imperative to acknowledge and explore the often-overlooked influence of obesogens. Imagine obesity prevention as a three-legged stool, with diet and exercise forming the familiar two legs. However, the third leg, representing obesogens, has been obscured from view and consideration for far too long. These chemical compounds disrupt the delicate balance of our normal metabolism, creating a ripple effect that extends beyond conventional lifestyle factors.

Obesogens wield the power to throw our metabolic processes into disarray. They interfere with the body's hormonal regulation systems, perturbing the delicate equilibrium that governs weight maintenance. This disruption predisposes individuals to weight gain and poses a formidable challenge to conventional weight management strategies. Understanding obesity solely through the lens of calories in and out becomes an oversimplification when chemical exposures also play a key role.

Recognizing the role of obesogens is not an attempt to diminish the importance of a healthy diet and regular exercise. Instead, it is a call to broaden our perspective and refine our strategies in combating obesity. In essence, the adage "you are what you eat" needs an extension—"you are what you're exposed to." As we grapple with the multifaceted nature of the obesity epidemic, acknowledging the influence of obesogens becomes paramount in constructing a more complete and impactful framework for public health interventions.

Mounting Evidence

The most recent evidence for obesogens comes from forty scientists writing in three review papers that cite 1,400 studies. After reviewing data from human cell and animal experiments and human epidemiological studies, the reviews cite nearly fifty chemicals as having obesogenic effects. The list includes BPA and phthalates—both plastic additives—a significant discovery since a 2020 analysis found a significant link between BPA levels and adult obesity in twelve of fifteen reviewed studies.[10]

The review also lists PFAS compounds, so-called "forever chemicals" or "persistent organic pollutants (POP)," as obesogens. Food packaging, cookware, furniture, and child car seats contain these compounds. How do these compounds impact weight gain? A two-year randomized clinical trial found that people, especially women, with the highest PFAS levels regained more weight after dieting.[11] And it's not just environmental pollutants, according to the review papers. For example, some artificial sweeteners, antidepressants, and triclosan, an antibacterial agent banned from some US use in 2017, have known obesogenic qualities.

Cause and Effect

Directly proving a causal link between a hazard and a human health impact is hard because we'll never have randomized control trials. It's unethical, not to mention illegal, to perform harmful experiments on people. We can't purposely expose pregnant women to suspected endocrine disruptors. But we do have sufficient epidemiological evidence quantifying the causal relationship between obesogens and obesity development within specific populations.

Are we rushing to conclusions on obesogens?

Given all the variables impacting weight gain, some people believe jumping on the endocrine-disruptor weight gain bandwagon is premature. They might argue that for packaged food, it is more important to worry about how much food is in the package than trace amounts of chemicals in the food packaging.

Here's where people get it wrong. It's not a single exposure to trace amounts of endocrine-disrupting chemicals that

---

continued

concerns me. It's the buildup. EDCs can stay in your body and cause cumulative effects over a lifetime. For example, many EDCs accumulate in fat, remaining for years and even combining with other EDCs or reacting with them. No one knows the effects of these mixtures on humans, but we have some evidence that they contribute to several health problems. One study examined whether EDCs might increase the symptoms of attention deficit hyperactivity disorder (ADHD). In this study, teen boys gave urine samples that were then tested for endocrine disruptors. The young men with more EDCs in their urine also displayed more notable ADHD behaviors.[12]

Researchers see connections between several other conditions and exposure to EDCs. Clear-cut evidence is lacking—and correlation doesn't equal causation—but research continues.

A good example might be tobacco smoking and lung cancer. Most of us know that smoking causes lung cancer. But what's the proof? In the 1950s, cigarette smoking increased rapidly, becoming more widespread. At the same time, lung cancer went from a rare to a more commonplace illness, and by the early 1950s, it was the most frequently diagnosed cancer in American men. While tobacco usage and lung cancer rates increased in tandem, there was still insufficient evidence to establish a clear connection between smoking and lung cancer.

Then, in 1952, two American researchers conducted a three-year-long cohort study and found that men with a history of regular cigarette smoking had a considerably higher death rate than men who had never smoked or only smoked cigars or pipes. They said smokers' higher death rates were primarily because of heart disease and cancer. And the cancer death rates were unambiguously associated with regular cigarette smoking. They wrote, "The death rate from lung cancer was much higher among men with a history of regular cigarette smoking than among men who never smoked regularly."[13]

We have ample evidence from numerous studies demonstrating causal links between regular cigarette smoking and increased death rates from both coronary artery disease and lung cancer. Similarly, we can confidently assert, based on equally robust evidence gathered from hundreds of studies, the existence of causal relationships between certain environmental compounds and obesity's development.

But how do obesogens affect humans?

As our knowledge of obesogens' effects in laboratory and animal models grows, questions about how these compounds affect humans remain unanswered, meaning we still don't have significant clinical data to determine acceptable chemical exposure levels. Since there's a lot of uncertainty, it's hard to know exactly when to intervene.

For pesticides, the United States Environmental Protection Agency (EPA) uses a standardized process to measure animal toxicity and estimate human exposure to determine if the compounds should be restricted or banned, and then acts on those assessments.

In 1976, Congress passed the Toxic Substances Control Act (TSCA), which for the last forty-eight years has been the principal law regulating chemicals found in products other than pesticides, food, and cosmetics.

When the TSCA was enacted, there were approximately 60,000 chemicals already on the US market, and an additional 62,000 widely available chemicals were exempted from regulation and grandfathered in. These chemicals were allowed to remain on the market without undergoing safety testing or regulatory scrutiny.[14]

In 2020, scientists compiled a global inventory that uncovered over 350,000 chemicals and chemical mixtures authorized for commercial production and use, a significantly higher number than previously estimated. While the EPA oversees most chemical regulations in the US, the jurisdiction for food additives and packaging materials, including plastics in bottles, falls under the US Food and Drug Administration (FDA). Despite this oversight authority, the EPA has yet to prohibit any chemical under the TSCA. Presently, tens of thousands of compounds have evaded safety testing because the law was enacted after their market introduction. The TSCA merely mandates that manufacturers provide information about new chemicals released to the public, encompassing their environmental impact. The United States Court of Appeals even overturned the asbestos ban, citing insufficient cost-benefit analysis by the EPA.[15] In light of such challenges, the prospects for comprehensive regulations on the myriad other compounds still in circulation appear uncertain, highlighting the TSCA's current limitations as an effective regulatory framework.

The EPA has a specific program for testing endocrine-disrupting chemicals. The Endocrine Disruptor Screening Program (EDSP) uses a two-tiered approach to screen pesticides, chemicals, and environmental contaminants for their potential effect on estrogen, androgen, and thyroid hormone systems.

The true cost of hormone-disrupting chemicals to the healthcare system is a complex topic, as it involves factors such as the prevalence of exposure, the severity of health outcomes, and the effectiveness of regulatory measures. However, conservative estimates say hormone-disrupting chemicals add $340 billion annually to US healthcare costs.[16] Assessments of the financial toll do not address the pain, suffering, and other consequences associated with diseases resulting from chemical exposures.

There's been some progress, but it's slow, and government inertia rules the day. For example, the FDA banned BPA in baby bottles and sippy cups a decade ago based on much less science than we have now. However, this ban wasn't the result of government regulation. Instead, consumer concern and media attention fueled industry change—ultimately, the FDA insisted on a ban. Of course, these consumer campaigns aren't perfect—BPS and other bisphenols that replaced BPA are also estrogenic, toxic to embryos, and persistent in the environment. So, the changes were transient.

Think about the power of employers, schools, and companies as force multipliers. For example, two major supermarket chains recently insisted that their food packaging providers swap out all buffet containers because they contain thyroid-disrupting perfluoroalkyl acids.[17] That decision was driven by a study finding these chemicals in five—yes, five—containers.

Policy and transparency are critical. Ingredient information—from what's in products to what we know about the effects of these chemicals—starts a discussion about tradeoffs. Without basic information about chemicals in cosmetics and personal care products, researchers can't even sort out the effects to guide consumers.

There's still very little regulation requiring companies to disclose all their product ingredients and any potential side effects. Industry trade groups lobby politicians to block such regulation. In 2020, California enacted the Fragrance and Flavors Right to Know Act, a law mandating comprehensive disclosure of toxic fragrances, flavors, and ingredients in cosmetics, personal care items, and professional salon products to California's Safe Cosmetics Program database. According to the law, companies had to start reporting toxic fragrance ingredients beginning in January 2022.[18] However, such regulations are few and far between. Often companies just label their products with the word "fragrance" as an ingredient, even though that fragrance or scent can be made of dozens of endocrine-disrupting chemicals.

Although most obesogen research points to these substances' role in obesity or metabolic disruption, the effects are not always consistent, partly because tests, exposure doses, and model systems vary. BPA has stirred much debate over whether studies on fat cell precursors in culture or non-human animals can predict what happens in people. Although the FDA safety tests new chemicals, there are no randomized, controlled clinical trials to examine the effects of environmental substances on obesity or any other metabolic condition.

However, observational studies continue to support the idea that obesogens can similarly affect humans. Several years ago, a physician named Leo Trasande collected data from an extensive national survey of children on levels of BPA in urine and BMI. The study found a link between higher BPA levels and obesity. In the least exposed group, just one in ten was obese.[19] Meanwhile, in every other group, one in five was obese. That's what I'd call a sizable effect.

Other studies have found a relationship between BPA and obesity. Among Chinese children, preteen girls with higher BPA levels in their urine are more likely to be in the heaviest category. However, it's important to note that BPA metabolizes quickly, so a one-time urine sample doesn't reveal a person's lifetime exposure. Because these are only observational studies, we're left with a tautology. It's impossible to determine if the exposure or the condition came first.

Human data on other obesogens are even rarer. For example, a systematic review of studies on phthalates' potential link to obesity came up short when the researchers couldn't find enough methodological consistency across studies.[20] Indeed, scientists don't have quality assays to measure some of these substances in relevant tissues. In the 1990s, professor R. Thomas Zoeller at the University of Massachusetts Amherst found that polychlorinated biphenyl (PCB) affects thyroid hormone action in fetal rats' brains.[21] Given the similarities between human and rat thyroid receptors (they're structurally identical), it's safe to assume that Dr. Zoeller's findings apply to humans. However, he had no way of proving it. You can't measure thyroid hormone activity in people's brains. And measuring hormone activity in the blood—as is typically done—doesn't tell us anything about what's happening in the brain.

However, even as better biomarkers become available, getting solid, long-term data on the relationships between pollutants and human obesity is expensive, time-consuming, and ethically fraught. This reality leaves the obesogen field on the periphery of clinical practice and environmental policy. Even today, I rarely hear people in the clinical obesity medicine community talk about obesogens' contributions to extreme weight gain.

In animal models, we can show how chemicals increase weight and fat and some mechanisms by which this happens. Still, without more robust human evidence, it might be difficult for the healthcare community, and the public, to accept chemicals as significant contributors to the obesity epidemic.

Even if physicians had obesogens on their radars, given their ubiquity and persistence in the environment, there's very little they could do to limit or treat exposure in their patients. However, these realities give us even more reasons to study them.

What I want to avoid is nihilism. Environmental compounds are everywhere and in everything, but with acceptance comes the opportunity to understand the health damage they can wreak and at least make a dent in the problem.

Talley's Take: Lubriderm® Syndrome and the Case of the Sidelined Surfer

Ever since he could remember, Cliff wanted to be a pro surfer.

He grew up in Santa Cruz, California—renowned as one of the nation's top surfing towns.

After years of training and thousands of hours in the chilly Pacific, Cliff finally achieved his dream and became a regular competitor on the World Surf League's Championship Tour, a showcase for the world's top surfers.

Contrary to what you might see in the movies with the stoned surfer archetype, professional surfers are disciplined athletes who follow a strict training and dietary regimen. For the uninitiated, surfing is very much its own universe. It involves throwing yourself at Mother Nature's mercy, battling sharks, weather, the mighty ocean, and perhaps the most challenging opponent—yourself. So, preparation is paramount.

Even among this group, Cliff stood out. He trained hard—sometimes up to eight hours a day—to prepare his body for the rigors of his chosen sport. Besides strength training, pro surfers also increase their endurance with cardiovascular exercise. Cliff cross-trains by running, biking, paddling, or swimming for one to two hours, six days a week. He also sleeps up to twelve hours daily, which isn't uncommon for a world-class athlete.

Cliff had no problem with the physical training and strict diet. He enjoyed it. So, he was more than a little alarmed when his performance dropped. Accustomed to finishing first or second in most events, Cliff started consistently coming in seventh or eighth. He couldn't figure out why. Of course, it's natural for an athlete's performance to drop as he gets older, but Cliff was only twenty-five, and surfers compete well into their thirties. Also, Cliff hadn't changed his training routine or varied his strict diet, which was Mediterranean-style fare consisting of fish, whole grains, vegetables, legumes, fruits, nuts, seeds, herbs, and spices. Given his rigorous training schedule, we also had Cliff on several nutritional supplements since it was hard for him to take in enough nutrients.

After meeting with Cliff for over an hour and reviewing his latest lab results, I admit I was still at a loss. However, one thing stood out: Cliff's sex hormone-binding globulin (SHBG) level was off the charts.

Sex hormone-binding globulin is a protein that affects the functioning of sex hormones, including testosterone and estrogen. SHBG binds to specific sex hormones, removing them from direct circulation. In the bloodstream, sex hormones are found in two forms: free and bonded. SHBG is one of those molecules to which testosterone and estrogen bind. Another is the protein albumin. In contrast, when sex hormones bind to SHBG, they're inactive and have minimal—if any—biological impact on the body until they're released.

SHBG levels fluctuate as we age, starting high in childhood and falling at puberty's onset, between ages nine and twelve for most people. Cliff's SHBG level was much higher than we typically see in a man. Excessively high SHBG is problematic primarily for males and athletes because it decreases the amount of free testosterone. High levels of SHBG are associated with infertility, a decreased sex drive, and erectile dysfunction. Cliff's levels were so high that his body determined that it needed more estrogen. He was morphing into a pre-pubescent boy.

I still didn't know why this was happening. So, I started asking questions to see if Cliff was doing anything that might cause his SHBG to spike. Often when I see hormonal changes like this, I consider everyday products a cause. Cliff used Lubriderm® lotion five to six times daily to prevent his skin from drying out after long days in salt water. Lubriderm® contains parabens and phthalates, which can adversely affect reproductive hormone levels (luteinizing hormone, free testosterone, sex hormone-binding globulin), anogenital distance, and thyroid function. Parabens are a common ingredient added to many lotions to extend their shelf life. Manufacturers also like parabens because they affect the estrogen-like fatty layer under the skin, eliminating wrinkles. Phthalates are added to personal care products, including body lotions, to help lubricate other substances in the formula and to carry fragrances.

To see if Lubriderm® might be at the root of Cliff's problems, we tested four other professional surfers who followed a similar regimen of covering their bodies with lotion throughout the day. To no one's surprise, they all had elevated SHBG levels and comparatively little free testosterone.

So, in this case, the solution was simple: We eliminated the lotion and replaced it with a paraben- and phthalate-free alternative. We immediately saw improvements in Cliff's biomarkers, including his free testosterone level, which returned to what we'd consider a normal range for a twenty-five-year-old professional male athlete.

The main takeaway here is that diet and exercise alone might not be the main culprits when our bodies don't do what we want or perform as expected. It's not just about calories in versus calories out. If eating a little less and exercising a little more were all it took to lose weight, then weight loss would be as simple as grade-school math.

But if you've ever followed a diet program and achieved less than your desired result, you probably asked yourself, "What did I do wrong?"

The fact is you probably didn't do anything wrong. Just as the EDCs in Cliff's lotion made him sick, the same toxic compounds in the foods we eat are good at making us fat. That's one reason why weight-loss advice may not always work. In fact, even strictly following the best traditional advice won't lower your obesogen exposure. See, an apple a day may have kept the doctor away 150 years ago, but if that apple now comes coated with chemicals believed to promote obesity, then that advice is way out of date. In fact, apples have been named one of the most pesticide-laden produce choices out there.

The obesogen effect suggests that exposure to these chemicals, even at low levels, may interfere with the body's metabolism and fat regulation, leading to weight gain and difficulties in losing weight.

Regarding traditional dieting practices, it's essential to note that the effectiveness of any dietary approach can vary among individuals due to various factors, including genetics, metabolism, lifestyle, and environmental influences. While choosing certain foods like lean proteins, fish, fruits, and vegetables can benefit our overall health and weight management, the obesogen effect may indeed play a role in how our bodies respond to different dietary choices.

However, it's important to keep in mind that the research on obesogens is still in its early stages, and more studies are needed to fully understand their impact on weight regulation and how they interact with different dietary patterns. When it comes to weight management, a holistic approach that includes a balanced diet, regular physical activity, limited toxic compound exposure, and considering individual needs and preferences is likely to be the most effective strategy.

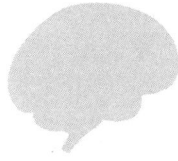

CHAPTER 6

Stuffed and Starving—Too Much Fat, Too Little Oxygen

You might wonder why a board-certified internist and pulmonologist specializing in critical care medicine is writing a book about obesity. It's a reasonable inquiry; the answer will become evident as you read this chapter. However, before addressing this question head-on, I'd like to familiarize you with lung physiology and how it interrelates with heart functioning.

To Air Is Human—Why do we need oxygen?

If the average person were asked about oxygen's essential purpose, they would probably answer, "for breathing." And that's true, but it's only a partial answer. We can't live without oxygen for more than a few minutes (permanent brain damage begins after four minutes without oxygen, and death can occur just four minutes later). The average adult brain consumes about 20 percent of the body's energy, and its primary function—processing and transmitting information through electrical signals—eats up a lot of resources. The brain's energy needs require a lot of oxygen.

Oxygen fuels our cells, combining with nitrogen and hydrogen to produce proteins that build new cells. When oxygen combines carbon and hydrogen, you get carbohydrates—our bodies' primary fuel source. We call this process cellular respiration. Oxygen is also critical for optimal immune system functioning. Low oxygen levels (hypoxia) can suppress some immune system responses.

The Lungs and Oxygenation

During my first year of medical school, my physiology professor offered a concise and correct explanation of lung function. He said in a thick Italian accent, "The good air, she's-a go in, and the bad air, she's-a go out." This description is a good starting place since the lungs' primary function is the exchange of oxygen for carbon dioxide, with oxygen-rich air inflating the lungs. In contrast, carbon dioxide, a waste gas, moves from your blood to the lungs, where it's exhaled (breathed out). This process is called gas exchange.

Gas exchange happens in the lungs between microscopic air sacs, the alveoli, and a network of tiny blood vessels in the alveoli walls. Each of us has about 480 million alveoli in our lungs. When you breathe in, the alveoli expand to take in oxygen. That oxygen passes into the blood. When you breathe out, the alveoli shrink to expel carbon dioxide.

But this process depends on all these healthy alveoli inflating and deflating with each breath. As you are likely aware, this requires that your diaphragm (the muscle separating the chest and abdominal cavities) move down to make room for the air-filling lungs. If this isn't possible, the bottom part of the lungs may not fully inflate, resulting in these alveoli being closed for business. If all works as designed, oxygen is extracted from the blood by our tissues, and this deoxygenated blood heads back to the heart and lungs to restore its oxygen supply—a straightforward, elegant concept.

The Heart's Role

Before discussing how oxygen and obesity interact, some critical physiological facts need to be cleared up. The bluish blood returning from the body for its oxygen refill first goes into the right atrium (the holding chamber) in the right side of the heart. Next, the blood goes into the right ventricle (the pumping chamber), which sends this deoxygenated blood to the lungs. The pressure needed to do this is a relatively low 10–20 mm Hg. This pressure is inconsequential compared with the pressure facing the muscular and robust left ventricle, which pumps blood into the body via the aorta with a pressure of around 120 mm Hg. The left ventricle wall is three times thicker (8–12 mm) than the right ventricle, which is comparatively thin at 3–5 mm. The left ventricle's function accounts for this thickness difference. It pumps oxygenated blood around the entire body, while the right ventricle only pumps blood to the lungs, a much shorter distance. Because the left ventricle pumps the blood further, it must generate more force during contraction, something it does with its added muscle power. Also, the blood pumped to the lungs from the right ventricle must be at lower pressure to prevent damage to the many thin capillaries in the lungs.

We get a sense of the left ventricle's power when we gauge our arteries' blood pressure (BP)—a measure of the ventricle's strength. A BP of 120 over 80 is ideal. We cannot directly measure pulmonary artery pressure, which takes blood from the right ventricle to the lungs, because there's no access. So, we use ultrasound or insert catheters to do this.

When the pulmonary artery pressure gets above 30 mm Hg, the right ventricle experiences pumping difficulties, something we see in patients with moderate to severe pulmonary hypertension. The right ventricle balloons, and this increase limits the left ventricle's filling ability.

Now that you have a background on lung physiology and its relationship to the heart's function, let's return to how a pulmonary and critical care physician became so profoundly interested in obesity.

José's Dilemma

About twenty-five years ago, I consulted on a case involving José, a thirty-year-old admitted to the intensive care unit with respiratory failure. José weighed over 400 pounds then, and this was not his first rodeo.

José's physicians were convinced he was in heart failure—a chronic, progressive condition marked by the heart's inability to pump or fill adequately. However, the cardiologist who examined José and studied ultrasound images of his heart told the attending physician that his heart was "great." The cardiologist performed an echocardiogram (a heart ultrasound), concluding that the left ventricle was contracting normally. In addition, the efficiency measurement, often called the ejection fraction, a measure of the percentage of blood the left ventricle pumps out with each contraction, was near 70 percent, well within the normal range. The only abnormality was some "stiffness" of the left ventricle, a condition known as diastolic dysfunction. Diastole refers to the phase of the heartbeat when the heart muscle relaxes, allowing the chamber to fill with blood. During diastolic dysfunction, the heart muscles stiffen and can't relax properly. So, the left ventricle fills with less blood, and less blood is pumped out.

"You don't need me," the cardiologist told the attending physician. "The heart is fine. What you need is the pulmonologist." From that day on, I realized garden variety cardiologists are left-heart doctors who pay little attention to the workings of the right ventricle and pulmonary arteries.

José's pulmonary artery pressure was 55 mm Hg—nearly three times normal—so the cardiologist suggested the attending physician consult me.

José's course was rocky, and although he made it through that hospitalization, I learned some months later that he died during a second bout of respiratory failure. Though José's other doctors couldn't explain his second episode of respiratory failure, by then, I'd already formulated my hypothesis about the connection between José's weight and his respiratory problems.

Role Reversal: Becoming the Teacher Again

I spent the first ten years of my medical career as an assistant professor at the UC San Diego Medical Center. Later, in 2020, I trained bright and eager nurse practitioners who joined my practice group. Like me, they saw how poorly our heaviest patients fared in the face of severe infections, blood clots, and traumatic injuries compared with normal-weight patients. Their hearts seemed to fail in every case, despite the cardiologists' reassurances that everything was "just fine." I reminded them that the heart specialists were discussing left ventricle contraction. If a ballooning right ventricle limited the filling of the left ventricle, then each contraction, as powerful as it might be, was ejecting smaller and smaller amounts of blood. This isn't a good situation!

These patients all had one thing in common. They had a long history of obesity, accounting for their "extreme physical limitations."

Severe leg swelling (edema) made walking more than a city block a Herculean task. The physical limitations showed left ventricle dysfunction; the edema signaled that the right ventricle couldn't overcome the pulmonary artery's high pressure, what we call "right heart failure."

Of course, I knew why this was all happening. However, the groundwork for all these phenomena was laid out years earlier, during my training period at UCSD.

The NOTT Enlightenment

During my fellowship training and for a few years afterward, the National Heart, Lung, and Blood Institute (a part of the National Institutes of Health) undertook a major study looking at the benefit of using 24-hour-a-day oxygen versus just nighttime oxygen in patients suffering from low oxygen levels.[1] Alveolar hypoxia—where the tiny air sacs in the lungs don't get enough oxygen—is common in chronic obstructive pulmonary disease (COPD) patients. I know this is hard to imagine, but in the late 1970s, there were no oximeters—small, noninvasive devices that estimate the amount of oxygen in your blood. Routine oxygen saturation measurements were unavailable, so drawing blood from a peripheral artery—a tedious and excruciating process—was the only way to measure oxygen levels. Talk about the dark ages.

The prevailing thought, particularly by those entities footing the bill, was that using oxygen for short periods at night would suffice in managing these patients. Thus, we started the Nocturnal Oxygen Therapy Trial (NOTT).[2] Unfortunately, and to no one's surprise, the study ended well before its expected completion date. The patients receiving only nocturnal oxygen were faring poorly compared to those receiving 24-hour-a-day supplemental oxygen. There were premature deaths and unexplained complications, and many years later, we learned that patients with morbid obesity fared the worst.[3]

Today, I'm sure that every reader of this book knows about sleep apnea. You likely know a friend or family member using a CPAP device—a continuous positive air pressure sleep machine. However, when the NOTT started, sleep medicine was still not a recognized branch of pulmonology or neurology. However, it didn't take long for some centers, including UCSD, to realize the importance of understanding sleep physiology. The combination of my background and these experiences transformed my fascination with obesity into a deep obsession.

The Sleep Apnea Connection

We've known for years that excess body weight is strongly related to frequent adverse breathing events in people with sleep-disordered breathing. There's a direct, predictable relationship between sleep apnea and obesity. Over 70 percent of all sleep apnea patients are severely or morbidly obese, and nearly 90 percent are overweight or obese.

The concern with this patient population revolves around the development of anatomical changes. These changes encompass an enlargement in neck circumference and the size of the glottis, a narrow slit-like valve regulating airflow in and out of the respiratory passages. This is attributed to redundant tissue in the upper airways and around the head and neck regions. This excess tissue obstructs the upper airways. Also, the excess weight compromises the diaphragm's ability to descend into the abdominal space.

Meanwhile, fat accumulation below the diaphragm impedes full diaphragmatic lowering, leaving many alveoli unexpanded. As a result, these patients see a drastic oxygen saturation decrease.

We consider an oxygen saturation level lower than 90 percent to be hypoxemia. Over the past twenty-five years, we've accumulated more data about reduced oxygen saturation in obese people. Given our discussion above, this makes sense. Obesity is associated with the visible fat we see and with omental or visceral fat that lies inside the abdominal cavity and surrounds the intestines. Fat accumulation under the diaphragm impedes the diaphragm's descent and the lungs' full expansion, meaning many alveoli never inflate. The recumbent sleep position magnifies this phenomenon, leading to low blood oxygen saturation.

While we know excess body weight correlates with frequent adverse breathing events in people with sleep-disordered breathing, the extent to which body weight contributes to blood oxygen desaturation has not been determined. However, obese patients experience more severe blood oxygen desaturation during sleep apnea episodes.[4]

Researchers examined 750 patients, aged thirty to sixty-two, from the Wisconsin Sleep Cohort Study, checking them for oxygen saturation, sleep duration, and other characteristics. Researchers observed 37,473 breathing events. Obese patients accounted for 40 percent of the cohort but contributed 62 percent to breathing events, with a mean oxygen desaturation of 4.8 percent. BMI was positively associated with oxygen desaturation severity, independent of age, gender, sleeping position, baseline oxygen saturation, and event duration.

As for the potential mechanisms linking obesity with oxygen desaturation, the researchers said that excess body weight reduces lung volume. In addition, the study results reinforce the importance of excess weight as a risk factor for sleep-disordered breathing development, progression, and severity.

In 2021, a study published in the *International Journal of Obesity* looked at various groups of obese individuals with and without obstructive sleep apnea (OSA). These data showed that the group of patients with Class III obesity (BMI greater than 40) and OSA had the lowest oxygen saturation. In contrast, the patient group with Class I obesity (BMI 30–35) and no OSA showed only mild hypoxemia. Of most interest to our discussion is the fact that those patients with Class III obesity and no obstructive sleep apnea had oxygen levels only slightly higher than the group with both Class III obesity and OSA.[5] The message is that obesity alone can lead to real-life hypoxemia.

Hypoxemia and Pulmonary Artery Pressure

Your blood oxygen level, or blood oxygen saturation, is the amount of oxygen circulating in your blood. Low blood oxygen content can cause shortness of breath, confusion, headache, and restlessness. After just 30–180 seconds (about 3 minutes), low blood oxygen levels can lead to a loss of consciousness. Many severe, even life-threatening health conditions result from hypoxia. For example, hypoxia in a finger or a toe can trigger gangrene. Likewise, hypoxic heart muscle can cause heart muscle death or myocardial infarction.

It has been known since the 1960s that chronic hypoxemia, a persistent lowering of the blood's oxygen content, can lead to increased pulmonary artery pressure. Clinical studies have shown that this phenomenon occurs over several years in those who live at high altitudes, where the partial pressure of oxygen in the air is reduced. Animal studies, primarily performed in chickens, demonstrate hypertrophy of the muscles in the lung's smaller arteries (arterioles).

In the 1970s, Dr. Talmadge E. King Jr. and his colleagues discovered that even short periods of hypoxemia, typical of OSA patients, increase the severity of pulmonary artery constriction. Dr. King and his colleagues induced hypoxemia in animal models by decreasing the oxygen percentage from 21 percent (normal air) to 10 percent—a dangerous state resulting in nausea, vomiting, lethargic movements, and sometimes unconsciousness. Following Dr. King's pioneering work, other experiments have shown that hypoxic periods increase the number of muscle cells in the artery wall, a process known as remodeling. We see this same phenomenon in the chicken experiments discussed above.[6]

The result is as expected. Brief periods of hypoxemia—typical of morbidly obese individuals and, to a lesser degree, people with Grade 1 or 2 obesity—can lead to elevated pulmonary pressures via blood vessel remodeling.

What I Call "Lethal Obesity"

Putting all this information together, we see why patients such as José have trouble coping with any slight perturbation in health status. Physical injuries (fractures), infections (such as SARS-CoV-2), or even minor surgical procedures can turn deadly. The longer someone is obese, the higher the chances of them experiencing multiple intermittent hypoxemia episodes.

The consequences of this are apparent. First, higher pulmonary artery pressure strains the right ventricle, which is thin and relatively weak as a pumper of blood into the lung, where the pressure is usually 10–20 mm Hg. When the right ventricle can't pump efficiently, it gets larger, eventually impinging on that all-important left ventricle—the one with all the pumping power delivering blood throughout the body via the aorta. As I stated earlier, an enlarged right ventricle limits the ability of the left ventricle to fill (diastolic dysfunction).

These patients, usually those with a BMI of 40 or greater, must deal with chronic hypoxemia. They have high pulmonary artery pressures (pulmonary hypertension) and all the complications above. A slight change in their condition, requiring the heart to respond by increasing its efficiency and pumping power, will be met with heart failure.

I call this type of extreme adiposity "lethal obesity," and the recent SARS-CoV-2 pandemic showed us just how important it is to avoid this condition.

And That's Only the Beginning

As discussed earlier, fat tissue, particularly adipocytes, produces bioactive molecules called adipocytokines. One of these is leptin, which helps control satiety. Other molecules, including tumor necrosis factor and resistin, increase low-density lipoprotein (LDL) production in human liver cells and degrade LDL receptors in the liver. Yet another fat cell derived hormone, resistin, accelerates arterial LDL accumulation, increasing the risk of heart disease. Obesity disrupts all these hormones.

Work from Japan's Osaka University published in the *American Journal of Physiology* in 2007 demonstrated that although there is a modest increase in fat cells in obesity, there is a much more significant increase in the actual fat cell size in obese people. At most, oxygen can diffuse about 100 micrometers inside a cell. So, as fat cells enlarge in obese subjects, they become hypoxic because the oxygen levels are dropping.

In the Osaka study, researchers could detect this fat cell hypoxia in obese mice by measuring partial oxygen pressure within the cell. As the cell's oxygen levels dropped, there was a corresponding decrease in hypoxia inducible factor (HIF-1Alpha), a small peptide that responds to the cell's changing oxygen supply. The gene controlling this peptide is downregulated. This peptide, when present, increases the blood supply to fat cells, so it should come as no surprise that in this study, there was also hypo-perfusion (a decrease in blood supply) of the fat cells that correlated with this oxygen decrease.

In these obese mice, this cellular oxygen decrease did not occur in their liver or muscle cells, where perfusion remained normal. Only in fat tissue did the perfusion decrease.

The decrease of oxygen in fat cells that uniquely occurs in obese mice comes from fat cell expansion that outstrips the cell's blood supply. This finding must be true, the researchers surmised, because muscle and liver cell oxygen levels, which they also measured, didn't drop. Only the fat cells suffered from low blood flow and low oxygen levels. We know these same effects occur in humans thanks to sophisticated imaging techniques, including PET scans.[7]

Along the same lines, a Turkish research group showed in 2017 that as oxygen delivery to fat cells decreases, these cells' metabolic activity decreases, contributing to a down-regulation of adiponectin, which, in turn, promotes insulin resistance. This was shown previously in vitro (in a laboratory using cell cultures), where human fat cells saw the changed expression of 1,300 genes that had been subjected to hypoxia.[8] In the Turkish experiment, there was not only a decrease in adiponectin but also an increase in leptin.[9] These two studies explain why diseases such as insulin resistance, diabetes, and coronary artery disease progress faster in obese individuals.

To be fair, data from published articles show that fat cells may adapt to decreased oxygen by slowing down their metabolism.[10, 11] But most of the research in this area suggests that enlarging fat cells are "sick," meaning they're not getting enough oxygen, resulting in a decrease in the activity of multiple genes, including those responsible for adiponectin coding. So, thanks to this work, we know it isn't just inflammation that makes obese fat sick. These cells also need more oxygen.

The Broader Consequences

Data show that many types of cancers are more prevalent in obese individuals. In addition, some large studies have suggested that certain malignant tumors are more aggressive in obese patients. An article recently published in *Frontiers in Oncology* showed that when fat cells hypertrophy, become hypoxic, and secrete the HIF I mentioned above, there is a corresponding loss in breast cancer estrogen receptors (ER).[12] Since many newer and effective drugs target these ER to attach to the tumor and kill cancerous cells, these ER-deficient tumors are harder to treat. So, sick fat cells can mess things up for the cancer patient.

In chapter 7, I discuss a subgroup of obese people who lack the metabolic risk factors typically linked with extreme body weight. Researchers from the UC San Diego and Washington University compared these patients with metabolically unhealthy non-obese, lean, and obese patients. They measured the amount of oxygen inside the patients' fat and liver cells in all three groups. They then assessed these three groups for inflammatory markers showing decreased insulin sensitivity and atherosclerosis.

In short, these markers would favor quicker development of diabetes and atherosclerosis (heart attacks, strokes, vascular insufficiency to the legs). As you might predict, the lean and healthy groups barely had any markers. However, both obesity groups, metabolically healthy and unhealthy, had significantly elevated markers.[13] This all means that obesity inevitably leads to low oxygen in fat cells, potentiating a host of reactions that hasten the development of life-altering diseases.

Some Final Thoughts

Maybe now it's becoming clear why, as a pulmonologist and specialist in critical care medicine, obesity interests me. However, putting the pieces in place to understand the oxygen-obesity connection took me years. Most of you reading these words have never heard of the oxygen-obesity relationship. Like epigenetics, oxygen is one piece of the obesity jigsaw puzzle. Knowing that anyone who is obese is at elevated risk for hypoxia, which causes a cascade of health problems, will hopefully clear up some mysteries about the disease's origins while showing why obesity is challenging to treat and manage.

I want to be clear that my goal in this chapter—as it is in every chapter—isn't to make people feel bad. As I told a patient recently, I'm not here to fat shame; I'm here to fat inform. However, I won't sugarcoat either. The eminent physicist Richard P. Feynman once said, "The first principle is that you must not fool yourself, and you are the easiest person to fool." If you don't understand the problem, anyone can delude you into believing you can be obese and metabolically healthy. However, with the right information, you might outsmart obesity. What could be better than that?

Obesity and COVID-19—
Flip Sides of the Same Coin

I never imagined seeing a pandemic in my lifetime, but SARS-CoV-2, the virus that caused COVID-19, changed everything. As I was outlining this book and considering how to outsmart and perhaps reverse obesity's ravages, a real-life experiment unfurled before us. From the pandemic's outset, obese people were doing far worse than their normal-weight counterparts.

Indeed, obesity is an established, independent risk factor for SARS-CoV-2 infection and for a patient's progression, once infected, to severe disease and death. Reasons for this increased vulnerability range from impaired breathing and cardiac dysfunction to altered immune responsiveness.

Though not all obese patients with severe COVID-19 require mechanical ventilation, many do because they develop acute respiratory failure. Obesity is associated with a higher risk of developing severe respiratory symptoms and complications, such as acute respiratory distress syndrome (ARDS), which usually requires mechanical ventilation. However, not all obese patients will progress to this stage, and some recover from COVID-19 without the need for mechanical ventilation. The decision to use mechanical ventilation is based on a combination of factors, including the patient's overall health, the severity of their respiratory symptoms, and the available treatment options.

A ventilator uses positive pressure to push air into the lungs to get oxygen into the body. The result is an increase in pressure inside the chest cavity. This pressure change comes at a price, impeding blood flow—a conundrum critical care physicians face every minute of every day while caring for obese COVID-19 patients. This disadvantage contributes to a well-documented increase in morbidity and mortality in this patient population.

Indeed, a recently published analysis of worldwide data showed that in every age group, SARS-CoV-2 viral infection was deadlier in obese individuals. For example, data culled from over 17 million people in the United Kingdom during the pandemic's early months found that simply being overweight (BMI 26–29) increased critical illness risk by 44 percent, and people with a BMI over 30 saw their risk jump to 97 percent.[14]

Other issues compound these mechanical problems. I review these here so you fully understand what we've already discussed in this book and how it applies to this once-in-a-lifetime pandemic.

Clotting Issues

COVID-19 changes clotting mechanisms because the virus injures endothelial cells, which respond by activating the body's coagulation system.[15] Add obesity to the mix, and the clotting risk escalates. The relationship of obesity to deep vein thrombosis risk—clots that occur in the lower extremity veins—has been known for decades. Less physical activity results in less muscle contraction and slower blood return from the legs, a situation favoring sludging and clotting. Many people who died from acute COVID-19 had signs of blood clots in their lungs, which had broken off from the legs and obstructed blood flow to the lungs. Of course, this hindered the exchange of oxygen and carbon dioxide.

Inflammation

In chapter 2, I make the case that obesity is a low-grade chronic inflammatory state, with an increased release and action of cytokines operating at a low but measurable level.

The earliest researchers looking at SARS-CoV-2 cited that the low-grade inflammatory state that naturally exists in obese people could only fan the flames, so to speak, of the cytokine storm accompanying SARS-CoV-2 infections.

But a 2022 Stanford University study provided a more direct reason: SARS-CoV-2, which causes COVID-19, can directly infect fat tissue. That, in turn, cooks up a viral replication cycle within resident fat cells, causing pronounced inflammation in immune cells residing in fat tissue. The inflammation converts even uninfected "bystander" cells within the tissue into an inflammatory state.[16]

A 2020 meta-analysis published in the *Journal of Medical Virology* found a clear-cut disadvantage for obese patients. As in the previous study, researchers explained that the best explanation for the apparent SARS-CoV-2 "enhancement" in this patient population was obese individuals' inflammatory state.[17]

Immune Factors

Obesity also weakens the immune system. Fat cell–secreted cytokines negatively affect immune cell production and storage. Data from both animal and human studies support this notion, suggesting that coronavirus vaccines may be less effective in obese and overweight people.

There is a connection here with vitamin D. It is a known fact that obese individuals have lower vitamin D levels than normal-weight people. This turned out to be a handicap. A recent study—based on data from Israel's first two coronavirus waves—found that people with a vitamin D deficiency were more likely to develop a severe or life-threatening case of COVID-19 compared with people who had sufficient vitamin D blood levels. Indeed, patients with vitamin D deficiency were fourteen times more likely to have a severe or critical case of COVID-19. The mortality rate for those with low vitamin D levels was 25.6 percent, compared to 2.3 percent among those with adequate levels.[18]

Vitamin D supports the body's immune system, enhances immune cell functioning, and inhibits inflammation that would increase COVID-19's severity.

The COVID-19–obesity connection should now be apparent. A new virus creates a robust inflammatory response, and obese individuals' more abundant and larger fat cells trigger what amounts to a five-alarm fire. Respiratory failure ensues, leading to intubation and positive pressure ventilation. Cardiac function falters, causing the heart and other organs such as the brain and kidney to be under-perfused, meaning they don't get adequate blood flow, which can lead to organ failure. Now you know why obesity is an independent risk factor for severe COVID-19 disease and death.

Talley's Take: The Vegetarian Paradox

My client Fred is forty-five years old. He's witty, successful, and pleasant. He's also a loving husband and doting dad. Fred's no different from many other middle-aged men, with one notable exception. He has trouble breathing.

"My doctor said something about obesity hypoventilation syndrome, but I'm not sure what he's talking about," said Fred.

Fred's diagnosis made sense and was unmistakable. Obesity hypoventilation syndrome (OHS), also known as Pickwickian Syndrome after Fat Joe, whom Charles Dickens described in *The Pickwick Papers* as a "wonderfully fat boy" remarkable for his "glorious appetite" and who had "many attacks of sleep during the day," was first described in the medical literature in 1956. However, the disease has probably been around much longer.

OHS is a breathing disorder usually seen in people with morbid obesity (BMI 40+ and at least 80–100 pounds overweight), leading to low oxygen levels and too much carbon dioxide in their blood. Hypoventilation—not moving enough air in and out of the lungs— creates the low oxygen and high carbon dioxide dynamic. People with OHS may also have problems sleeping because of obstructive sleep apnea.

Unfortunately, at six feet two and 325 pounds, my patient Fred fits the morbid obesity bill. He has all the classic symptoms— hyperhidrosis, tiredness, joint and back pain, difficulty breathing, sleep apnea, snoring, breathlessness, and high blood pressure.

However, it was Fred's breathing difficulties that concerned me the most. The lack of oxygen was putting added strain on Fred's heart.

"How did this happen to me?" said Fred during our weekly appointment. "I was a pretty active kid."

"We don't fully understand OHS's causes. It could have something to do with your brain struggling to control your breathing. But if I can speak candidly, Fred, I think the excess weight is the biggest issue here."

I don't know if Fred appreciated my response, but I had to be honest. Fred's weight was putting his life at risk. The excess fat on his neck, chest, and abdomen made deep breathing difficult and may have been producing the hormones somatostatin, dopamine, and neuropeptide Y, all of which depress breathing. Elevated neuropeptide Y can also stimulate food intake, decrease calorie burn, and increase fat storage.

Fred became a client after seeing Dr. Lonky, who was the first person to diagnose his OHS. The diagnosis was easy based on Fred's medical history, sleeping habits, BMI, and oxygen and carbon dioxide levels, which we measure with an arterial blood sample. Also, a finger pulse oximeter can approximate the blood's oxygen content.

Sometimes, a physician will also order a chest x-ray and pulmonary function tests to rule out other causes. A sleep study, called polysomnography, is sometimes used as well. For example, people with OHS often, but not always, suffer from severe sleep apnea. In addition, specialists may use a sleep study to test the possible therapeutic effect of continuous positive airway pressure (CPAP).

During our blood work on Fred, we also saw elevated suberate, ethylmalonate, and adipate levels, not uncommon with elevated CO_2. Ethylmalonate, adipate, and suberate give us information about a person's ability to process fatty acids. Adipate, suberate, and ethylmalonate elevations indicate metabolic blocks. When we use the three in combination, it usually shows carnitine deficiency. Carnitine levels can be deficient in either blood or tissue (usually muscle) or both.

Carnitine, or L-carnitine, derives from an amino acid and is the generic term for several compounds. The brain, liver, and kidneys make it, and it's naturally present in many foods—especially foods of animal origin—and is available as a dietary supplement. In addition, it plays a vital role in energy production and fatty acid metabolism.

The normal blood levels in humans are 50–60 µmol/L for total carnitine and 40–50 µmol for free carnitine. Unfortunately, Fred's carnitine levels were far below these baseline numbers.

Primary carnitine deficiency can cause severe medical problems, including severe brain dysfunction (encephalopathy), a weakened and enlarged heart (cardiomyopathy), confusion, vomiting, muscle weakness, and low blood sugar (hypoglycemia).

As Fred and I discussed his diagnosis and health, I discovered something I hadn't known before. On a friend's advice, he'd recently switched to a vegetarian diet. Because he'd given up all animal products—carnitine's only source—he wasn't getting the carnitine his body needed.

Fred would need a lot of treatment, including a comprehensive diet and exercise program, but I suggested he add some grass-fed beef. People often ask about the difference between grain- and grass-fed beef. What does it mean?

Cattle are ruminants, meaning their diets must contain forages such as grass and hay. They graze plant material that humans cannot eat. Most cows start their lives the same way. Calves are born on pasture and stay there until weaned. In the traditional model, ranchers finish cattle by feeding supplemental grains, like corn, soybeans, and wheat, to increase their energy intake.

Grass-fed animals have lifetime access to a pasture and are not fed grains. In nature, cattle would never encounter grains. It's much better for them, and for us, to avoid grains. Grass-fed beef has less fat and is usually lower in calories. It's also higher in Omega-3 fatty acids than grain-fed beef, which may help prevent cardiovascular disease.

Along with healthy amounts of grass-fed beef, which Fred was happy to add to his diet, OHS treatment involved weight loss and treatment of his sleep-related breathing disorder. Sometimes, weight loss corrects many symptoms and problems, such as obstructive sleep apnea. However, given Fred's weight and overall health, we knew he'd need more to treat his OSA. So, Dr. Lonky prescribed CPAP or noninvasive ventilation. This device delivers air through Fred's mask whenever he sleeps or naps. CPAP delivers air at a constant pressure both when you breathe in and when you breathe out.

Because OHS can cause serious health problems, sometimes surgery is needed (e.g., gastric bypass surgery) to help with weight loss, which eventually happened for Fred since he found it hard to control cravings on his own.

Today, I'm happy to report that Fred is down more than 100 pounds and has kept that weight off for more than two years.

It wasn't easy, and Fred admits that the old habits surface occasionally. However, for the first time, he knows he's on the right track, and it's showing up in all the right places, including on the bathroom scale.

SECTION
II

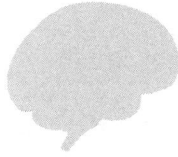

CHAPTER 7

Fat Chance—Why You Can't Be Healthy at Every Size

Is beauty synonymous with goodness?

At first glance, this notion might appear implausible, yet there was a time when such a belief held sway. In ancient Greece, the concept of *kalokagathia* guided lives—a Platonic doctrine that linked outer beauty with a beautiful mind and virtuous character. The German philosopher Immanuel Kant identified an appreciation for beauty as a sign of one's inclination toward a morally upright nature.[1]

Even today, the beauty-is-good stereotype permeates our culture. We assume that clear skin, sparkling eyes, a symmetrical face, and hair that shimmers in the sunlight equate to intelligence, sensitivity, competence, and kindness. It's also why we trust celebrities, even if we suspect some of them are nuts.

The tendency to "judge a book by its cover" also includes forming opinions based on body weight. "Fat people are lazy." "They lack willpower and self-control." "If they didn't eat so much, they wouldn't have health problems." For millions of people, fat stigmatization is a part of daily life.

I'm not breaking any new ground here by saying we shouldn't judge people based on their weight or body size. However, fat shaming isn't just immoral; it doesn't work. A University College–London study found that people who experience day-to-day weight discrimination gain weight.[2]

Scales don't measure human worth. Losing weight is hard for most people, and for folks who are obese, it's a Sisyphean task. I don't know anyone who can't get behind these ideas and doesn't view fat shaming as reprehensible. That's the easy part.

Here's where things get trickier. I will not, under any circumstances, go in the opposite direction and "bless" obesity. What do I mean by that? I don't support the notion that you can be "healthy at every size"—because evidence shows that you can't. Don't believe me? Well then, see for yourself.

Dispelling the Urban Myth of Metabolically Healthy Obesity

Have you ever heard of the term "metabolically healthy obesity," or MHO for short? It seems like an impossibility. Yet, it's become fashionable in recent years to say just that. It means that while obesity increases the risk of developing insulin resistance (leading to diabetes), atherosclerosis, cancer, and dozens of other acute and chronic illnesses, a person who is obese may not necessarily develop these problems.

Is this true? The answer, like obesity itself, is complicated. However, one thing is clear: Metabolically healthy obesity is a medical misnomer. How do we know? Because we have ample evidence that you can't be simultaneously obese and healthy.

In a 2017 study published in the *Journal of the American College of Cardiology*, researchers examined 3.5 million electronic health records—categorizing them by body mass index and whether a person had diabetes, high blood pressure, or high cholesterol. The research team classified about 15 percent, or slightly over half a million people, as obese and metabolically healthy.

Now, here's the rub. Over a five-year follow-up, those obese people who did not have diabetes, high blood pressure, or high cholesterol at the outset were 49 percent more likely to develop heart disease, 7 percent more likely to have a stroke, and 96 percent more likely to develop heart failure. In absolute terms, the heart disease increase was about one extra case per 1,000 people, which might seem like nothing, but it is significant when you apply it to the total medically healthy obese population of 500,000 (about half the population of Montana). Then, the number jumps to 500 people.

In this study, obesity increased long-term heart disease risk. It's also important to note that common heart disease risk factors—diabetes, hypertension, and cholesterol, which are typically found in people who are obese—carry a much heavier disease burden. (A disease burden refers to the total cumulative impact of a health problem on a given population.) Having one, two, or all three of these diseases increased the number of cardiac events by five cases per 1,000, seven cases per 1,000, and ten cases per 1,000.[3] That's a lot.

A unique yet interconnected British study observed over 400,000 individuals over a span of more than ten years and discovered that metabolically healthy obese (MHO) individuals experienced a higher occurrence of heart failure and respiratory disease incidents compared to individuals with a normal weight. Furthermore, the research indicated that in comparison to metabolically healthy but not obese participants, individuals with MHO faced elevated rates of new-onset diabetes, atherosclerotic cardiovascular disease

(ASCVD), respiratory disorders, and all-cause mortality. These findings imply that MHO individuals might possess a lower risk of cardiovascular and respiratory issues than those who are both obese and metabolically unhealthy. Nonetheless, their risk remains higher than that of metabolically healthy non-obese individuals, particularly when it comes to heart and respiratory failure diseases.[4]

I can cite other studies, but they all reach similar conclusions: obese but metabolically healthy people are at higher risk of metabolic and respiratory diseases than normal weight individuals.

METABOLICALLY HEALTHY OBESITY WITH CARDIOVASCULAR DISEASE IN COMPARISON WITH ALL-CAUSE MORTALITY

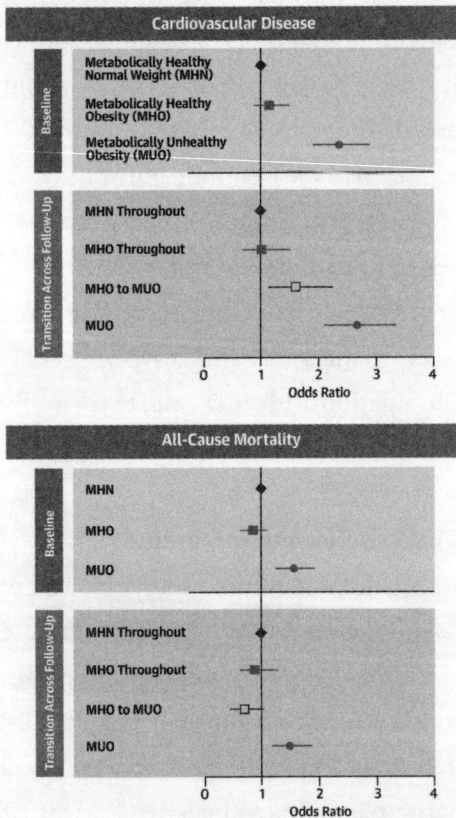

Graphic credit: *Journal of the American College of Cardiology.* Used with permission.

Don't Cling to the Fairy Tale

So, if the data show that you can't be healthy and obese, why do some people still cling to this fairy tale? The problem, I believe, is that we've become seduced by the fact that a small percentage of obese people (between 3 and 22 percent) have normal metabolic profiles—healthy blood pressures, good lipid and inflammatory profiles, and high insulin sensitivity at a specific time.[5]

That last phrase—at a specific time—is key. Think of metabolically healthy obesity as a Kodak moment. It's a snapshot in time that captures an obese person when they might not have any obvious weight-related medical problems. However, the good times won't last. Most people with metabolically healthy obesity become unhealthy within three to five years.[6] They're still at increased risk of heart disease, stroke, and other health problems. Metabolically healthy obesity is akin to a kid who seldom brushes and flosses his teeth and eats a lot of candy but still has no cavities. Trust me; the cavities are coming. It's just a matter of when. Thus, no one who is obese is perfectly healthy. Even those in the "metabolically healthy" category live on borrowed time.

So where do we go from here? Instead of focusing on whether someone who is obese is healthy today, we should think more about the health problems they will inevitably face.

Do obese people live longer?

I hear the questions now. "Dr. Lonky, I read somewhere that obesity is protective and helps people live longer. So why are you saying they'll face problems down the road?" This person is asking about the so-called "obesity paradox," which, in an odd twist, suggests that fat might be protective. Indeed, extant evidence shows that obesity in older people and those with chronic diseases, particularly cardiovascular disease, may be protective and even decrease the risk of premature death. For example, a 2020 study found that overweight and Class I obese trauma patients had better survival chances than patients with a "normal" BMI.[7] A 2019 study by Italian researchers offered similar findings, concluding that being moderately overweight protects against several comorbid diseases as we age, making it a marker of a healthy aging process.[8]

However, consider this before you reach for that extra slice of carrot cake: The obesity paradox is a lot of baloney. Obese people live shorter lives than healthy-weight people and are at increased risk for at least sixty chronic and acute diseases.

And forget about these studies showing a health benefit of being overweight or obese. I'm aware of no major studies showing a survival advantage for obese and overweight people. Consistently, a normal-range BMI links to the greatest survival odds.

Not only is there no clear benefit to being either obese or overweight, but I'd also argue that fat isn't protective in any way. Indeed, three recent studies with large cohorts and long follow-up periods debunk the idea that fat may offer some protective benefits.

One of the studies, published in the *European Heart Journal*, compared cardiovascular disease (CVD) outcomes in 296,535 overweight and healthy-weight subjects. In total, 3.3 percent of women and 5.7 percent of men in the study experienced some sort of cardiovascular event. Subjects with a healthy BMI of 22–23 had the lowest cardiovascular disease risk. From there, an increase in BMI correlated to an increase in CVD risk. Researchers saw a similar risk for increases in waist circumference, waist-to-hip ratio, waist-to-height ratio, and body fat percentage.[9]

Obesity's Impact on Your Body and Health

I can't think of one aspect of health, from reproductive and respiratory function to memory and mood, that excess weight, especially obesity, doesn't diminish. Obesity affects every bodily system and its functioning. As an example, obesity compromises fertility by changing how a woman's body stores sex hormones. Fat cells convert a male hormone called androstenedione into a female hormone called estrone. Estrone is the weakest type of estrogen, but it's powerful enough to affect luteinizing hormone production. LH is a gonadotrophic hormone produced and released in the anterior pituitary gland that helps control ovarian and testicular functioning.

And it's not just the woman's weight that affects fertility. Obese men are more likely to have low or even nonexistent sperm counts—obesity can elevate body temperature, especially around the scrotum. It can also lead to hormonal imbalances. Obese men are more likely to have higher estrogen levels and lower levels of inhibin B and androgen, two sperm-producing hormones.[10]

Obesity is a known risk factor for bloodstream and soft tissue infections, pneumonia, and acute coronary syndrome, a term describing a range of conditions related to sudden reduced blood flow to the heart, including heart attack and unstable angina.

The message is clear: obesity is a risk factor for many chronic and acute illnesses. Even within the normal BMI category, disease risk increases beyond a BMI of 22–23. Conversely, the data consistently show that the leaner a person is, the lower the CVD risk. I'm not offering my opinion; I'm stating a scientific fact based on the best available data.

Don't Count On Exercise to Save You

And if you're obese or overweight, even an active lifestyle is not enough to counter the adverse effects of those excess pounds.

In one of the most extensive studies of its kind, researchers analyzed data from over 500,000 adults and grouped people based on activity levels and body weight. Then, they evaluated their heart health by assessing three major heart attack and stroke risk factors: diabetes, high blood pressure, and high cholesterol.

Study participants who were overweight or obese, regardless of their activity levels, were more likely to have high cholesterol, diabetes, and high blood pressure than their normal-weight peers.

"While being active was linked with better heart health . . . the results indicate that exercise doesn't compensate for the negative effects of excess weight," wrote the study authors, contradicting the popular notion that one can be "fat but healthy."[11] The study adds to existing evidence that there is no such thing as "healthy obesity," and any misconceptions about being "fat but fit" should be erased posthaste.

I'm all for health policies that promote physical activity and fitness. But weight loss must be prioritized as the goal for those who are obese or overweight.

Many people face challenges in achieving weight loss, and attaining a slim physique and low BMI may prove difficult, especially for those classified as overweight or obese. However, the data shows that losing weight—even just a few pounds—will improve your health.

So, I've laid out a compelling case for why you can't be healthy and obese. I described how being overweight, let alone obese, increases your risk for dozens of life-altering illnesses. But how did we get to where people say aloud that you can be healthy and obese? From where did this nonchalant attitude toward obesity's health risks originate? Fortunately, we don't have to look very far for answers.

Fat Acceptance and the Birth of a Movement

Fat Acceptance, more commonly known as Body Positivity, dates to the 1960s when the National Association to Aid Fat Americans (NAAFA) campaigned for equal rights for people of higher weights while offering some pointed criticism of the small but growing American diet industry.

Today, NAAFA goes by the National Association to Advance Fat Acceptance. But the NAAFA's mission remains unchanged—to encourage accepting and appreciating one's body, even if it is severely overweight. Fat Acceptance touts the virtues of "compassionate self-care" and "body diversity" while "challenging [the] scientific and cultural assumptions" about weight.[12] We see these ideals in department stores, beauty products, and exercise clothing line ad campaigns featuring models of many sizes.

Fat Acceptance has even made inroads into the world of high fashion. After decades of waif-like models, New York Fashion Week now features many "plus-size" women strutting down the catwalk. Dove has run several ad campaigns featuring plus-size models. Chrissy Metz, an actress who has struggled with weight issues, had a lead role on the hit NBC drama *This Is Us*, playing a character coming to terms with her large body.

The Fat Acceptance movement also champions body acceptance and empowerment in the "health versus weight" debate, encouraging obese and overweight people to shift their focus from losing weight to other healthy habits, such as eating whole foods and moving more, both laudable goals. Ironically, such healthy habits will produce weight loss and improve epigenetics, as I explained in an earlier chapter.

I understand the Fat Acceptance movement. It helps plus-size people cope with a world pitted against them and find a welcoming community that defies conventional medical wisdom about weight. Fat Acceptance offers people who feel ashamed and targeted a road map to self-acceptance.

The Fat Acceptance community raises some valid points.

1. Yes, the number on the bathroom scale gives an incomplete picture of your health.

2. As I discuss in chapter 2 about defining obesity, body weight and body mass index don't consider body composition.

3. Conventional criteria for healthy body weight are based on certain body types and may not be appropriate for everyone, particularly people of certain races and ethnicities.

4. Most people would agree that harassing or criticizing people about their eating habits doesn't work and often has the opposite of the desired effect.

Fat Acceptance and the Dangers of Groupthink

We all believe certain things and prefer associating with people who feel the same. They rarely challenge us since they share similar beliefs and values. They're our tribe. However, some tribes form around false or harmful beliefs and ideas. It doesn't matter how much information there is to the contrary, they don't want to hear it and will defend their beliefs to the end.

The Fat Acceptance movement manifests this intolerance. Indeed, it shares a censorious, tribe-like mentality toward anyone who says anything that remotely contradicts the belief that body size is unrelated to health.

Here's one example. In 2021, former British Prime Minister

Boris Johnson unveiled his "Better Health" campaign to combat obesity—a move prompted by his bout with COVID-19, which included a stint in intensive care he believes was brought about by his reported body mass index of 36.[13] However, many critics pounded Mr. Johnson's effort, citing its overemphasis on personal responsibility and underemphasis on obesity's root causes, which they incorrectly cited as poverty and inequality.

Nothing in Mr. Johnson's public pronouncements characterized obese people as lazy, weak-willed, or gluttonous. Yet, the hue and cry effectively derailed his efforts to raise awareness about the obesity-COVID connection in a country that would have benefited from the message, as recent data show that 62.8 percent of British adults are overweight or obese.[14]

As I see it, the problem with Fat Acceptance isn't a few dozen social media influencers and celebrities talking about being proud of their size. Nor would I object if the Fat Acceptance community consisted only of plus-size people celebrating their strengths and working toward common goals of better health and well-being.

But that's not what's happening. Instead, Fat Acceptance, like many insular movements, has become an echo chamber for its followers, many of whom live in denial about obesity's consequences, and can be a harmful source of misinformation. Fat Acceptance is self-acceptance taken to a dangerous level.

In 2020, Cancer Research UK, the world's largest independent cancer research organization, launched a campaign to raise awareness that obesity is the second modifiable cause of cancer after smoking. The backlash reverberated worldwide, with people from the Fat Acceptance community accusing Cancer Research UK of "fat shaming," and even petitioning to have the ad legally removed. The Fat Acceptance folks took offense because Cancer Research UK chose to raise awareness about the cancer-obesity link.

I read the "offending" ads. Cancer Research UK didn't point fingers or criticize any single person or group. The ads didn't say, "Fat people get cancer" or, "Being fat will give you cancer." Instead, the charity reiterated a research-backed, mainstream scientific fact: obesity is a known cancer risk factor. This is no different than saying, "Smoking kills." Does this mean that smokers are bad people or don't deserve medical treatment? Of course it doesn't. These are both campaigns designed to raise awareness. If they ruffle a few feathers along the way, that may be the price of saving lives.

Coming Back to Reality

I agree with anyone who insists that alongside a conversation about the health risks obesity poses, we need greater awareness of how weight stigma unfairly burdens millions of people.

Perhaps if more people realize and accept that obesity isn't a simple math equation, there will be a greater society-wide understanding of and empathy toward people with weight problems. Disassociating disease from the person living with it is no easy feat, particularly obesity since its outward manifestations are clear and hard to ignore.

I understand how even well-intentioned health messaging can be misinterpreted or misconstrued, creating even more problems. As a physician, I share these concerns. But where do we draw the line?

Direct messaging may sometimes hurt feelings, but we shouldn't ignore the risks obesity poses to human health, particularly if it means saving lives. In the 1970s, sensationalist anti-tobacco ads helped drive home smoking's dangers. Sure, there's still a hipster aesthetic to cigarettes, and for impressionable young people, an undeniable cool factor to smoking. But, by and large, the public is tuned in to smoking's many dangers. We must adopt a similar, no-nonsense approach toward obesity.

We should all be happy with ourselves and accept that no one is perfect and that all humans are works in progress. But we should be equally vigilant about not spreading misinformation. There should be an end to attempts to normalize body sizes that increase a person's disease risk and decrease their lifespan. Most importantly, we shouldn't feel that talking about specific topics is *verboten* if that conversation could help save lives. The research is unambiguous about obesity: if you carry excess body fat, you're putting your health at risk—if not today then certainly in the future.

It's crucial to approach obesity with empathy and compassion. I celebrate the efforts of people who seek a world where all bodies are valued and respected, and yes, there's more to health than body weight. Health isn't a moral virtue, and fatness isn't offensive.

But we must balance our feelings with messaging and tangible solutions that make a difference in people's lives. It's dishonest to perseverate over the social stigma while ignoring obesity's side effects. Fat shaming is reprehensible; however, I won't go to the opposite extreme either. I will not, as I said earlier, bless obesity.

I realize that some of you reading these words will not believe what I said about obesity. You may genuinely believe that a person can be healthy at every size. And you'd be right if being at a larger size didn't increase your risk of severe illness and death. But, at some point, you must face and accept objective reality. You can't be healthy at every size because that's what you've decided, or been conditioned to believe, or because some celebrity or Instagram guru says you can.

Sorry, but that's not how it works. That's why I've tried to give you the facts about obesity. Accepting obesity as OK is not wise. But, with knowledge, we can outsmart it.

Talley's Take: Why You Can't Be Healthy at Every Size

"Chris, I'm nervous. The Emmys are just a few weeks away, and I'm a bloated mess."

Elaine, a TV personality and businesswoman, was anxious about being ready for the major industry event. In addition, she'd recently given birth and, like many women, was carrying excess weight.

None of this was abnormal, and I shrugged off her concerns. "You look fine. You just had a baby, and you're right where you should be," I said.

"No, I can't show up looking like this. You know my public image revolves around my body," Elaine responded, growing impatient that I was dismissing her concerns.

Dr. Lonky discussed obesity's serious health consequences in this chapter. However, it's important to note that the opposite end of the spectrum can also be harmful. Trying to lose weight too quickly or becoming dangerously underweight likewise presents dangers to one's health. This is the other side of the coin that the chapter looks to shed light on.

I counseled Elaine on avoiding anything radical and just sticking with the post-pregnancy program we designed. The goal was to exercise moderately daily and eat a Mediterranean-style diet with lots of protein. She planned to eat sweet potatoes, quinoa, lean meats, and healthy fats including limited quantities of avocados and olives.

Sadly, when Elaine left my office that day, I knew she wouldn't follow my advice. She wouldn't take any chances with hundreds of people taking her picture and publishing it across millions of TV and computer screens. "The internet lives forever. I don't want someone to show me a photo five years from now of me at my heaviest weight," she said before leaving. I decided not to mention that she had weighed 30 pounds more while pregnant. Still, I knew Elaine would eventually learn that you can't be healthy at every size, even if that size is a two.

Like many people in the entertainment industry, Elaine is part of a group I refer to as the "hungry days crowd." Depending on their desperation level, they will schedule days or weeks to starve themselves before a big event or role. I have an actress client who cuts off contact with the outside world on days when she knows she will starve herself.

Some actors go through extreme weight loss for movie roles. Award-winning actor Adam Driver shed 50 pounds for his star turn in the movie *Silence*. Multi-talented Anne Hathaway dropped 24 pounds to play Fantine in the movie adaptation of *Les Misérables*. But these actors lost weight under careful medical supervision for a short time to fit specific roles.

What I saw with Elaine, and so many others in the entertainment industry, was a willingness to sacrifice their health and well-being to look good regularly. It's an open secret that Hollywood doesn't treat male and female actors equally regarding looks. Male actors are celebrated for losing and gaining significant weight for parts. The industry encourages female stars to lose weight even if they don't need to because it's part of the deal in Tinseltown. They love to post Instagram photos with a quote about loving the "unfiltered photos" of their bodies. But somehow, they conveniently leave out the part about how they cry themselves to sleep.

The irony is that the more the women starve themselves, the harder it is for them to lose weight. Sure, extreme calorie restriction can help you drop weight quickly, but it's not an effective method if you want to keep weight off long term.

Your body will conserve energy when you restrict calories. It does this by slowing down your metabolism so that you don't burn off fat and calories as quickly. Starvation causes an increase in the hunger hormone ghrelin, and a decrease in the satiety hormone leptin. Ghrelin levels are higher in obese people, and these levels increase when these folks lose weight.

Caloric restriction, which today takes the form of intermittent fasting, may also raise LDL (bad) cholesterol levels by altering metabolism from glucose to ketones. This transition prompts the body to utilize lipids instead of storing them. As lipids exit cells, they circulate in the bloodstream and enter the liver for conversion into ketones. Caloric restriction may also create critical nutrient deficiencies.

Here's the bottom line: The more you restrict calories to lose weight, the more your body will protest. Depriving your body of what it needs will only make long-term weight loss more challenging and put your mental and physical health at risk.

Here's what I'd do instead: lose weight sustainably and healthily.

Again, I love the Mediterranean diet because it's excellent for weight loss but doesn't require a drastic calorie restriction. The Mediterranean diet is beneficial, reducing morbidity and mortality in people with cardiovascular risk.

Eat a balanced diet with lean protein, fruits, and vegetables, and drink plenty of water. Getting enough rest and physical activity are also essential to maintaining your weight or safely losing weight. While exercise isn't great for weight loss—you can't outrun a lousy diet—it's helpful for weight maintenance.

I also recommend to clients that they eat regularly throughout the day. This is the best way to avoid mindless snacking. Eating breakfast is especially important since it gives your body nutrients and starts fueling your body for the rest of the day. In addition, eating lots of fresh produce, like a variety of fruits and vegetables, will provide your body with many vitamins and minerals. These foods can help support your weight-loss goals.

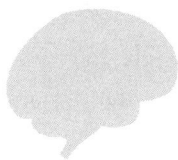

CHAPTER 8

Open All Night—How the 24-Hour Food Environment Impacts Obesity

U nless you live off the grid, it's impossible to ignore the seismic shift that has happened in the American food landscape over the last twenty years. Today, we inhabit a world of massive portion sizes, relentless food advertising, and the easy accessibility of ultra-processed, calorie-dense, and inexpensive food options. Food is at every venue imaginable, including drugstores and gas stations. Big box stores like Costco, BJ's, Wal-Mart, and Target sell groceries. Add to this the list of 200,000 fast-food restaurants, drive-in windows, convenience stores, vending machines, and food courts, and suddenly everywhere you go, you have no choice but to see that food is plentiful and cheap. Not to mention, companies spend millions on marketing and advertising to keep us eating their products. So, let's get real: the modern food environment unintentionally sabotages weight-loss efforts for millions of people.

One way to think about your food environment, says Kelly Brownell, director of Duke University's World Food Policy Center, is to ask yourself this: "How far are you from a doughnut?

How close are a Dunkin' Donuts, coffee shop, supermarket, or 7-Eleven that sells doughnuts?"[1]

Not only do we eat poorly, but we also eat mindlessly. In his book *How to Eat*, Thich Nhat Hanh wrote, "Spend time with your food; every minute of your meal should be happy."[2] In Japan, "enjoy your meals" is a foundational dietary directive. Similarly, in the much-studied "Blue Zones"—those regions of the world known for having a high number of centenarians and a lower incidence of age and lifestyle-related diseases—people typically practice mindful eating by sitting down and savoring their meals rather than eating on the go or in a rush. But how many of us do this?

In fact, we do the opposite. We eat without conscious awareness or attention to our surroundings, a big change from just a few years ago. When I was growing up, my brothers and I never ate in the car unless it was food our mother packed for a long trip. We had three meals a day and maybe a snack. Most nights, we sat down to family dinners. Today there are no prescribed mealtimes or locations, and people eat all day. With food delivery services, online ordering, and the rise of mobile apps, we now have access to a wide variety of food options, no matter where we are. We eat practically anywhere, anytime.

Availability isn't the only problem. Look around. Food companies employ various marketing and advertising strategies to incentivize and encourage consumers to eat their products. These tactics are designed to create demand, increase sales, and foster brand loyalty. But what they do, more than anything, is stimulate craving and increase overconsumption. This isn't a minority view. Charles Courtemanche, director of the Institute for the Study of Free Enterprise (ISFE) and associate professor of economics at the University of Kentucky's Gatton College of Business and Economics, says America's rising obesity rates are due, in considerable measure, to a nonstop barrage of eating incentives. The ISFE's data show that a combination of supercenters (massive supermarkets), warehouse clubs, and restaurants contribute significantly to obesity's rise.[3]

Along with greater access and more incentives, our food composition has changed. Processing typically alters food's nutrient value, taste, texture, smell, and appearance. Scientists design highly palatable foods to maximize consumption, engineering them in ways that make it difficult to put the brakes on eating. These foods hijack the brain, subverting personal decision-making and leading to health problems, obesity being the most obvious. It's not hard to figure which foods trigger overeating. When was the last time you binged on squash? But guess what? If squash were crunchy and salty—known appetite triggers—you'd probably overeat it.

Designed for Disease: How the 24-hour Food Environment Fuels the Obesity Epidemic

Did you know the average person makes at least two hundred daily food decisions? One study found that the average person made 226.7 food-related decisions each day. The number was even higher for the study's obese participants who made over one hundred more food-related decisions daily than overweight people.[4] That's a lot. While some people may believe that food choices are entirely within our control, research in psychology and behavioral economics has shown that many food decisions—like a thousand other decisions we make daily—are automatic and influenced by factors beyond our conscious awareness. They're part of what I refer to as "mindless eating." If you're at a party or other social event where food is being served, you'll keep eating from a bowl of chips or nuts well past the point of satiety simply because they're within arm's reach. The result is that we consume five hundred more daily calories than we did in the 1970s.[5]

The next question to ask is, Why are we consuming more calories today and making more daily food decisions than we did in the past? The first answer is that in the 24-hour food environment, we have more choices available to us. Availability stimulates consumption. When food is at hand, people are more likely to consume it even if they are not necessarily hungry or in need of additional calories, a phenomenon known as the "availability heuristic."

Convenience is another factor driving consumption. When food is easily accessible and requires minimal effort to obtain, people are more likely to indulge in it. And that's not all. In the 24-hour food environment, visual cues are everywhere. Seeing food can trigger cravings and stimulate hunger, even if you've just finished eating. Larger portion sizes, which follow increased availability, can also lead to overeating. The more you have on your plate, the more you'll eat, sometimes without any awareness of the extra calories you're consuming. The food industry's investment in marketing reinforces and reminds us of this constant availability, making it hard to resist the temptation to consume certain foods.

The psychological perception of scarcity can also play a role. When people perceive a particular food as rare or limited, they may feel compelled to consume more when it becomes available. This principle also works in economics. As Robert B. Cialdini observed in his textbook *Influence: The Psychology of Persuasion*, "Opportunities seem more valuable to us when their availability is limited."[6] In this case, we're talking about the opportunity to eat.

Understanding availability's impact on consumption is particularly vital for promoting healthier eating habits. Increasing the availability and accessibility of healthier food options while reducing the influence of unhealthy choices can positively influence our dietary choices and overall health.

The Biology of Eating: A Daunting Complexity

Everyone knows the word "appetite," but how many people can define it? I view it simply as a person's desire to eat. It's distinct from hunger, the body's biological response to a lack of food. A person can have an appetite even if their body isn't craving food. Many factors cause our appetite to rise and fall, leading us to eat less or more than our bodies need.

Research shows we're less discriminating about what we eat when we are hungry. But conversely, many variables increase our appetites, such as anxiety, stress, boredom, memory, habit, conditioning, and of course, our environment. Biology plays a major role in eating. We eat to survive. So, it makes sense to pay attention to physiological cues indicating hunger, and not be seduced by appetite alone. But what exactly are these cues?

Early researchers believed that stomach contractions or growls—a sign the stomach is empty—triggered hunger. This theory explains why many weight-loss strategies were (and still are) based on "tricking the stomach" into thinking it's full. Receptors in the stomach and intestines play a significant role in detecting the presence of nutrients and signaling feelings of fullness. However, hunger is a complex physiological and psychological process involving multiple factors. The sensation of hunger is so powerful that it can still persist in people who have had their stomachs removed for medical reasons such as cancer. This phenomenon occurs because hunger is not exclusively driven by physical stomach contractions or nutrient detection. The process of hunger involves a complex interplay of hormones, neurotransmitters, and signals from the brain, which can still occur even if the absence of a physical stomach.[7]

Other biological hunger cues include biochemistry, glucose, and hormone levels. Here's how some of this works. When blood glucose levels drop, the liver can send signals to the brain that increase hunger. The liver, which stores glucose in the form of glycogen, breaks down glycogen back into glucose and releases it into the bloodstream, helping to prevent hypoglycemia (low blood sugar). As you can see, the liver plays a crucial role in maintaining blood glucose levels within a relatively narrow range. The brain detects a change in blood glucose through various mechanisms, including direct sensing of glucose levels and signals from other organs. The hypothalamus region in the brain responsible for regulating various physiological processes, including hunger and satiety, plays a central role in interpreting these signals. The brain then releases specific hormones and neurotransmitters that increase appetite and motivate you to seek food. The hypothalamus's influence is so profound that in rat and mouse experiments, animals with a damaged hypothalamus either gain a lot of weight or starve to death.[8] This finding tells us that the hypothalamus regulates the motivation to eat.

Insulin, a hormone produced by the pancreas, regulates blood sugar levels and energy storage. When you eat, especially carbohydrates, your blood sugar levels rise. In response to the increased blood sugar levels, the pancreas releases insulin into the bloodstream. Insulin helps cells absorb glucose from the bloodstream, which cells use for energy or store for later use.

When you are hungry and have not eaten for a while, your blood sugar levels tend to be lower. In this state, the pancreas reduces insulin secretion because there's less need to transport glucose into the cells since there's less glucose available from food. Instead, the body utilizes stored energy sources such as glycogen and fats to maintain blood sugar levels and fuel the body.

Leptin, often called the "satiety hormone," plays a crucial role in managing our appetite and energy balance. It works like this: When your body senses a decrease in leptin levels, it's essentially getting a signal that there aren't enough fat reserves available. This signal can result in you feeling hungrier and more compelled to eat.

Conversely, when your body has plenty of leptin, it tells your brain that there are sufficient fat stores, which in turn reduces your hunger and gives you a feeling of fullness after eating. So, when you lose fat or have lower leptin levels, your brain interprets this as a sign of diminished energy reserves. In response, your brain increases your appetite and hunger because it perceives an energy deficit.

Nature, Nurture, or Beyond: The Complex Factors Influencing Taste Preferences

Suppose you were to create a comprehensive list of your favorite and least favorite foods and the varying degrees of fondness or aversion you have toward each. The result would be a unique catalog that is entirely your own, like a fingerprint. However, unlike fingerprints, your taste preferences are not fixed; they evolve. While genetic and epigenetic factors form the biological basis for taste preferences, cultural conditioning, biological programming, family dynamics, and life experiences also play vital roles in shaping individual flavor choices.

Let's clarify some definitions. "Taste" commonly refers to "flavor," which is influenced not only by our taste buds but also by our sense of smell and texture. Humans can naturally detect five taste types: sweet, bitter, salty, sour, and umami (savory). However, our genetic and epigenetic makeup determines our sensitivity to these tastes. In contrast, our preferences for specific flavors are more subjective and influenced by past experiences and cultural attitudes toward food.

Our taste preferences undergo predictable changes as we age. For instance, we enjoy sweetness less as adults than in childhood.

On the other hand, our fondness for vegetables typically increases in adulthood when compared with our early years.

How can we explain these trajectories? In 2022, researchers identified around five hundred genes that directly influence our dietary preferences.[9] These genes encode proteins that detect taste sensations like sweet, salty, bitter, sour, and umami. Differences in these taste receptor genes can make individuals more or less sensitive to specific tastes, influencing their liking for or aversion toward certain flavors.

For instance, a specific variation in the TAS2R38 gene can heighten a person's sensitivity to bitter tastes, potentially making them less likely to enjoy foods like broccoli and Brussels sprouts if they carry this genetic variant. On the other hand, researchers believe that one reason for kids' fondness for sugar is the evolutionary advantage of seeking out calorie-rich foods to fuel their growing bodies, mainly when food is scarce. Of course, it is also possible that children simply love the taste of sugar, which adds to their preference for sweet foods.

Regarding vegetables, there's a reason why you, as an adult, have no problem ordering a salad for lunch, even though you probably went five rounds with your parents at the dinner table over broccoli when you were a kid. From an evolutionary perspective, humans and many other animals have developed an aversion to bitter tastes as a protective mechanism against accidental poisoning. Taste receptors known as TAS2Rs (Taste 2 receptors) mediate bitter taste perception. They're located on the tongue's taste buds and other mouth parts. However, today, we don't have to rely on taste receptors because we've largely identified which plants are harmful and which are safe to consume. Despite this knowledge, our aversion to bitterness persists, even though many bitter vegetable compounds offer crucial nutritional benefits.

So how do we get over that bitterness aversion to tolerate and even enjoy our greens? Mostly by just eating them. It's a type of immersion therapy where you become comfortable with something you don't like simply by repeated exposure. If you eat something enough times, you will grow to like or at least tolerate it. Part of it is social learning: we hate vegetables as kids; we see adults eating vegetables; we become adults and learn to like them, too. Another part of it is the simple fact that eating a certain food enough times will make it more appealing.

But the question that naturally follows is: Why does exposure eventually negate our dislike? We don't have a clear answer, but epigenetics may play a role in taste preferences, potentially surpassing the influence of genetics. For instance, studies have shown that a mother's diet during pregnancy can influence the epigenetic regulation of her children's taste-related genes, potentially affecting their taste preferences later in life. This happens because nutrition is an essential epigenetic modulator, influencing phenomena such as DNA methylation and histone modifications. These two major epigenetic mechanisms play crucial roles in regulating gene expression.

Nutrition can influence epigenetic processes through the availability of methyl donors and cofactors involved in DNA methylation pathways. For instance, folate, vitamin B12, and choline are essential methyl donors in the one-carbon metabolism pathway, which is directly linked to DNA methylation. A deficiency or excess of these nutrients in the diet can affect DNA methylation patterns and, consequently, gene expression.

Similarly, certain dietary components, such as polyphenols in fruits and vegetables, can affect histone modifications and gene expression. These compounds can interact with histone-modifying enzymes, leading to changes in the accessibility of genes and altering their expression patterns.

Studies have shown that a person's early-life nutrition can have long-term effects on their epigenetic markers and gene expression patterns, potentially influencing health outcomes later in life. Additionally, some research suggests that nutrition can reverse or mitigate epigenetic changes associated with specific diseases or conditions.[10]

An alternative explanation could be that each time we encounter a specific food, it gradually diminishes our inherent skepticism toward new things. It's natural for us to be cautious about novel items. A similar pattern can be observed in species like rats. They cautiously sample a small portion of something, observe the effects, and then gradually consume more. This gradual approach is also the basis for introducing new foods to our diets. It's not a conscious decision where you think, "This might be risky, Dr. Lonky." Instead, repeated exposure over time may gradually reduce this cautiousness.

However, in certain instances, simply repeating exposure might not suffice to overcome the strong aversion that arises when we associate a negative experience with a specific taste. This phenomenon is known as "conditioned taste aversion," and it has the potential to persist throughout our entire lives. For instance, a particularly unpleasant encounter with oysters on a single night could be sufficient to permanently deter you from consuming any shellfish in the future.

On the other hand, some taste preferences remain enigmatic, defying clear explanations. Take, for instance, my intense distaste for meatloaf despite having no recollection of any particularly traumatic experiences related to it. The origins of my meatloaf dislike are a mystery, as it cannot be attributed to social learning—my mother regularly prepared meatloaf for our family. Maybe I had a significant negative encounter with it during my early childhood, possibly falling ill shortly after eating it. Alternatively, it might be linked to my aversion to onions, as my mother always added them to her meatloaf, leaving a lasting negative impression that solidified into a persistent hatred over time. The reasons behind such taste preferences sometimes remain elusive.

In essence, even the tiniest experiences have the power to shape our food preferences in ways we might not consciously realize. Are you familiar with Marcel Proust's seven-volume masterwork *Remembrance of Things Past*, also known as *In Search of Lost Time*? When Proust's narrator, Marcel, eats the crumbs of a madeleine dipped in lime blossom tea, this sensory encounter acts as a catalyst, vividly resurrecting his past experiences and emotions, illuminating the intricate interplay between taste and memory. Imagine all of these memories triggered by just a taste of a cookie! It's easy to see how these engrained memories and associations can override cultural norms, evolutionary inclinations, and other influences. This complexity is one reason scientists find taste preferences challenging to comprehend fully.

Environmental factors play a vital role in molding an individual's taste preferences. Early exposure to diverse flavors, cultural influences, and dietary habits during childhood all contribute to shaping one's palate. As we encounter specific tastes repeatedly, we may develop a preference for them irrespective of genetic factors. For instance, growing up in a culture where spicy foods are prevalent can lead to a natural liking for spicy flavors due to early exposure.

Moreover, environmental cues significantly impact our food decisions. The psychological cues in our surroundings can trigger us to eat more, and the larger portions offered by food establishments may contribute to overeating. Research shows that people finish whatever is served to them, even if they aren't hungry or thirsty.[11]

The interplay of taste preferences involves a complex combination of genetics, epigenetics, and environmental influences. While genetic and epigenetic factors lay the groundwork, experiences and exposures throughout life play a substantial role in determining individual flavor choices. Epigenetics, in particular, shows promise as a significant factor in shaping taste preferences, but ongoing research is necessary to understand its relative impact compared to genetics.

Mexico: A Case Study

Mexico, which has the dubious distinction of having the world's highest childhood obesity rate and second-highest adult obesity rate (three-quarters of the population is now overweight or obese), is probably the best place to view the toxic food environment's effects. Mexico's tipping point, say many experts, traces back to the early 1990s when the country joined the North American Free Trade Agreement (NAFTA), paving the way for an influx of global fast food chains and making cheap, ultra-processed foods available everywhere.[12] In post-NAFTA Mexico, residents drink, on average, 163 liters of sugary soft drinks per person annually. The COVID-19 pandemic further exacerbated Mexico's weight problems by decreasing physical activity. Over 330,000 Mexicans have died from COVID-19, the world's fifth-highest recorded death toll, with obesity and high blood pressure as the chief underlying conditions complicating the disease.[13]

This alarming scenario underscores the complex interplay between trade policies, globalization, and public health outcomes. It highlights how international trade agreements such as NAFTA can have profound and lasting effects on a nation's health landscape. The prevalence of cheap, processed foods and the rise of global fast-food chains in Mexico serve as a stark example of how trade decisions can contribute to the escalation of obesity and related health issues.

Moreover, the COVID-19 pandemic unveiled the intricate relationship between existing health conditions and the severity of infectious diseases. In Mexico, where obesity and high blood pressure were prevalent pre-pandemic, COVID-19's impact has been particularly devastating, underscoring the importance of addressing both infectious diseases and the underlying health disparities and lifestyle factors that contribute to a population's vulnerability.

The Mexican experience serves as a cautionary tale and a call to action for policymakers, health professionals, and communities worldwide to collaboratively address the root causes of obesity and promote healthier lifestyles. Only through concerted efforts can we hope to mitigate the long-term health consequences of a toxic food environment and build a more resilient, healthier global society.

Cultural Conditioning: How Our Interpersonal Relationships Influence Eating Behavior

Who doesn't enjoy family gatherings, getting together with friends, and taking part in group activities? Such occasions are an opportunity to check in with each other, share ideas, and even lend social and emotional support.

The people closest to us—friends, family, and coworkers—also impact our food choices. Peer influence can affect food choices and preferences in children as young as age two. A published study shows that preschool-aged children model their peers' eating behavior. For example, when a vegetable-disliking preschooler was seated with a group of vegetable-loving students, the child was more likely to alter food preferences and eventually give vegetables a chance.[14]

If you've ever lived with teenagers, you understand the value they place on social acceptance. Fitting in and having a sense of belonging is vital to them. The social pressures teens experience significantly affect their eating behaviors. These influences are so powerful that they alter youth behavior, even supplanting parental and familial influences.

The family strongly influences the environment in which a child grows up. We've discussed obesity's complexity and manifold influences. While the obesogenic environment is broad and multifaceted, the home environment and parenting equally impact a child's dietary and physical behaviors. An *American Journal of Clinical Nutrition* study found that parental influence significantly affected young children's food selection. Parental monitoring or the threat of parental oversight led to young children choosing fewer unhealthy foods and foods with lower total caloric content.[15]

According to Duke University School of Medicine and the Duke Global Health Institute, kids whose moms encourage exercise and healthy eating and model these behaviors are more likely to be physically active and eat healthily. In the Duke study, researchers studied the relationship between the home environment and preschoolers' obesity-related behaviors, including their dietary and exercise habits. The researchers analyzed data from 190 kids, aged two to five, whose mothers were overweight or obese. First, they collected information on the children's food intake, classifying them as junk or healthy. Then, to gauge their physical activity levels, the kids wore accelerometers for a week, which measured moderate to vigorous physical activity and sedentary time.

The researchers also looked at the mother's socioeconomic factors, which did not affect their children's physical activity but influenced their dietary habits. The mothers also reported information about family food policies and physical activity levels, the accessibility of healthy versus junk foods, the availability of physical activity equipment, and whether they modeled healthy eating and exercise habits.

After analyzing the data, the researchers found significant associations between these environmental measures and pre-schoolers' physical activity and healthy versus junk food intake. They concluded that a healthy home environment and parental role modeling are essential to promoting children's healthy behaviors. The home environment influenced the children's dietary habits more than their physical activity levels.[16] This study reminds parents that their children observe and mimic both their good and bad behaviors. They watch and learn by observing what we do. The food preferences and eating habits they develop at home can, and often do, last well into adulthood.

Of course, providing a healthy home environment isn't easy for many families. Low-income families face barriers to healthy eating, possibly contributing to higher-than-normal obesity rates. One roadblock is that healthy foods such as vegetables, fruits, and whole grains are more expensive than less healthy foods. Another is time. Home-cooked meals require time, vigilance, and patience. Unfortunately, many folks, particularly single working parents, have less time and energy for meal preparation—and who can blame them?

How Food Advertising Influences Eating Behavior

In 1969, Congress passed legislation banning television and radio ads for cigarettes. President Nixon signed the bill into law, which took effect in September 1970.[17] Public health officials rightly argued that the ads caused people to smoke more and raised their cancer risk. Some public health advocates claim we should hold food companies to the same standards as cigarette manufacturers, arguing for tight regulations on food advertising since their products can cause weight gain and obesity. However, the burden of proof is higher for obesity than for smoking, partly because the impact of food on our health isn't cut and dried.

In 2008, the Federal Trade Commission (FTC) reported that the food industry in the US spends almost $10 billion per year marketing food and beverages that appeal to children and adolescents, including $1.6 billion to target them directly with soft drinks, fast food, and cereal promotions.[18] The Center for Science in the Public Interest claims food and beverage companies spend nearly $2 billion annually marketing food, much of which is unhealthy, directly to kids.[19]

Despite this widespread recognition of the negative impact of marketing unhealthy foods, the practice continues unabated. Dummies do not own food companies. These conglomerates use licensed cartoons, superheroes, and other popular entertainment characters to target young children with foods that horrify most self-respecting nutritionists. Healthcare professionals, parents, and politicians have called for industry and government regulation because food and entertainment companies don't police themselves. Efforts to develop voluntary, uniform nutrition standards for foods and beverages marketed to children have met with predictable and strong resistance from industry and have been stymied by Congress, which enjoys a far-too-cozy relationship with industry lobbyists.

Indeed, the advertisements we see may wield as much influence over our body weight as the dietary choices we actively make. Advertising amplifies brand recognition and subtly manipulates our decision-making processes. However, it's important to note that advertisements also frequently provoke heightened consumption levels, often taking viewers by surprise. A comprehensive meta-analysis conducted at Yale University, scrutinizing forty-five studies, established that up to 26 percent of the variation in eating behavior and eventual weight outcomes can be traced back to cravings and other responses elicited by food cues, especially those visually presented in commercials.[20] If food ads are that powerful, should we limit children's exposure to them? Some feel this is a topic worth considering.

Palate Priming

In a separate 2009 Yale study, leading obesity researcher Kelly Brownell and his colleagues designed a series of experiments to understand how food commercials embedded within a television program primed people to seek out snack foods unconsciously. Behavioral priming occurs when exposure to one stimulus (e.g., a television commercial) influences a response to a subsequent stimulus (e.g., a bowl of snacks) without conscious awareness or intention.

Researchers compared snacking behavior in two experiments before and after exposure to different commercials. To ensure the participants were unaware of food advertising's behavioral effects, they recreated an environment where food ads typically appear, such as a home den or bar. Also, the participants didn't know the researchers designed the experiment to measure advertising's influences on their snacking behavior.

Adding another layer of disguise, the snack food brands given to the participants were unrelated to those advertised on television. Researchers also eliminated the data collected from the participants who correctly guessed the experiment's fundamental purpose. The experiments occurred during similar times of the day, which helped control hunger. The television viewers also reported how hungry they were and when they had eaten last to help ensure ad-induced rather than hunger-related snack consumption.

The study found that the children consumed 45 percent more snack foods when exposed to food commercials. Adults exposed to snack food advertising also ate more. The researchers did not relate these snacking behaviors to conscious intention or reported hunger.[21]

Advocates for tight regulations on food advertising claim that our obesity epidemic is proportional to the unhealthy foods we see on TV and in other media outlets. But the burden of proof is high for such claims. And so far, the public health community's battle against food ads has been a losing endeavor.

Many industry critics argue that children are especially vulnerable to food advertising because they lack the experience and knowledge to objectively evaluate persuasive advertising appeals. They're also incredibly susceptible to suggestions, which all food marketers know. In very young children, research has found that for every one-hour increase in TV viewing per day, there are higher intakes of sugary beverages, fast food, red and processed meat, and overall calories (48.7 kcal/day).[22] Other research has shown that children who spend over three hours daily in front of TV or computer screens are 50 percent more likely to be obese than children who watch fewer than two hours.

Many US policy experts say they're not optimistic about the prospects of legislation restricting food advertising to children. "I really don't have a lot of hope for regulating food ads," said Robert Paarlberg, a Harvard-affiliated global food and agricultural policy scholar, in an interview with NPR.[23] I also have little confidence in the government's ability to regulate food ads. All advertising is commercially protected speech; a court must weigh in to overthrow these protections. Many years ago, the Obama administration proposed voluntary guidelines on food advertising. However, the White House dropped that proposal in 2012 after Congress passed a bill requiring a cost-benefit analysis of the guidelines and whether they would lead to food and beverage sector job losses.

In 2020, the food industry instituted the Children's Food and Beverage Advertising Initiative (CFBAI), a voluntary self-regulatory program to help companies shift advertising targeted toward young children to highlight healthier options.[24] While the member companies, including Coca-Cola, Burger King, and Mars, have made minor nutritional improvements to their products, they've done nothing meaningful to safeguard kids from unhealthy food and beverage marketing practices, according to a research report by the University of Connecticut's Rudd Center for Food Policy and Health.[25]

Indeed, efforts to cut back on marketing unhealthy foods to children have barely moved the advertising needle from junk food to genuinely healthy products. On average, American kids see three to five fast food ads daily. And about 50 percent of all ads directed at children are for food. According to a Federal Trade Commission report, food companies across the board spend less than one percent of their marketing budgets promoting fruits and vegetables. Conversely, Coca-Cola spends $4 billion annually on advertising. And no, cherry-flavored Coke doesn't qualify as a fruit.

Convenient Food, Inconvenient Weight Gain

Did you know that convenience stores can increase a person's obesity risk? Indeed, studies show that obesity increases proportionately with the number of convenience stores in each neighborhood. Community food environments and neighborhood stores can significantly influence a person's weight status.

In one study, researchers followed two groups of low-income and ethnic/racial minority children aged three to fifteen. The investigators assessed how changes in the number of food outlets at various distances from the children's homes affected their weight. They found an association between unhealthy childhood weight changes and increased numbers of convenience stores. For example, having an additional convenience store within a mile of a child's home over twenty-four months resulted in an 11.7 percent greater risk of a child being in a higher body mass index (BMI) range than other children of the same sex and age.

In contrast, having an additional small grocery store that sold healthy food items within a mile over twenty-four months was associated with a 37.3 percent lower risk of being in a higher BMI category.[26] Understanding the impact of local food environments on our weight and health became even more urgent during the COVID-19 pandemic.

In a separate study, researchers mapped food outlets across Mexico (fast food, convenience stores, restaurants, supermarkets, and fruit and vegetable stores) to investigate how the retail food environment affects adult obesity risk. Almost all (99.5 percent) neighborhoods had at least one convenience store, but less than half (42 percent) had a fruit and vegetable store.

In saturated urban neighborhoods, for every 10 percent increase in convenience stores, the average resident's weight increases by approximately 2.2 pounds, equivalent to BMI 0.4 units (kg/m^2) higher.[27] These study findings suggest that convenience store chains increasingly meet people's food needs instead of supermarkets.[28] This is an unfortunate trend.

Schools: The Great Home Lunch versus School Lunch Debate

Everyone, from politicians to public health officials, drones on about the necessity of providing kids with healthy food choices at school.

And why not? Just as employed adults spend their days at work, children spend much of their days at school. The US Department of Agriculture's School Lunch Program and related federal school meal programs serve breakfast, lunch, and after-school snacks to over 30 million children daily. That's a lot of food. Some research shows that taking part in school breakfast programs correlates with lower BMI, while lunch programs have no positive benefit. The authors of these studies opine that school breakfast programs may reduce obesity risk because they help spread food intake across many hours.

The next question is, are these government lunch programs all they're cracked up to be? Maybe not. One study found that a third of middle school students who regularly eat school lunches are overweight or obese. They're also more likely to have high LDL (bad) cholesterol. In the study, which compared kids who brought lunch from home versus those who ate school lunches, the latter group:

- Were more likely to be overweight or obese (38.2 vs. 24.7 percent)

- Were more likely to eat two or more servings of fatty meats like fried chicken or hot dogs daily (6.2 percent vs. 1.6 percent)

- Were more likely to have two or more sugary drinks a day (19 percent vs. 6.8 percent)

- Were less likely to eat at least two servings of fruits a day (32.6 percent vs. 49.4 percent)

- Were less likely to eat at least two servings of vegetables a day (39.9 percent vs. 50.3 percent)

- Had higher LDL cholesterol levels

The school-lunch kids were also less likely to take part in active sports such as basketball, moderate exercise like walking, or team sports than their home-fed counterparts. And they spent more time watching TV, playing video games, and using computers outside of school.

Recent data show that while about 30.6 million US students eat school lunches, only 6 percent of school lunch programs meet the USDA requirements. For example, the average sodium content was twice the recommended daily allowance, and 80 percent of schools exceeded the rules to keep fat to less than 30 percent of total calories.[29] While efforts have been made to improve school meals' nutritional quality, not all school lunch programs meet these requirements consistently. Compliance can vary based on factors such as funding limitations, infrastructure constraints, availability of resources, and local policies. Some schools may face challenges in meeting the nutritional guidelines due to budget constraints, limited kitchen facilities, or difficulties sourcing healthy food options.

Schools also sell food to students outside of the school meal programs. These foods and beverages can be purchased from school cafeterias, vending machines, and school stores, and are referred to as "competitive foods." It's believed that 50 percent of all US students today eat these competitive foods during a typical school day, a 20 percent increase from 2013–2014.[30] Most of these foods are high in calories and low in nutritional value.

I don't want to give the impression that I'm opposed to federally funded school meal programs. One million households with children are regularly "food insecure," meaning that families face "limited or uncertain access to adequate food," according to the United States Department of Agriculture (USDA) website.[31] Food insecurity correlates with poor health and wellness outcomes. Healthy nutrition, meanwhile, is crucial for students' learning.

In a 2019 literature review, University of Virginia researchers highlighted nutrition's critical importance to academic performance and cognitive ability.[32] The brain needs fuel to function correctly, and research continues to show that blood glucose levels can directly affect a human's ability to learn and process information. Deficiencies in specific nutrients, such as iron, can also negatively affect memory and learning.

As the obesity epidemic has grown, researchers and public health advocates have called for public policy efforts to address the toxic food environment in schools. Unfortunately, progress is slow. While it's clear that our food systems are contributing to the obesity epidemic, improving the global food environment presents many challenges. Taxing unhealthy foods and drinks, curbing junk food marketing, and realigning agricultural subsidies with health all sound great on paper, but they've proved hard to implement or haven't worked well in actuality.

Will that reality change soon? I'm hopeful, but I have concerns. As Cameron English, director of biosciences at the American Council on Science and Health, wrote in a recent op-ed, "There's an odd disconnect between the way we talk about the causes of obesity and the solutions we employ to help people manage their weight."[33] Indeed, recent results suggest we need a different approach.

Here's just one example. Since obesity translates from childhood to adulthood, we need to look no further than a September 2021 literature review examining efforts to reduce adolescent calorie intake. The authors collected fifty-two clinical trials published between 2009 and 2019. Each paper investigated "school-based interventions, community-based interventions, interventions through mass media, and food sector interventions."

Many of these interventions were educational (e.g., nutrition classes for parents and students). However, nine studies examined disruptive policies like school menu changes, increased physical activity during school hours, restrictions on TV food advertisements, and sugar taxes. Can you guess the results?

Overall, most of the intervention studies failed to show consistent effects on changing children's BMI. Many studies, mainly based on school interventions, did not show effective results.

The authors offered a handful of explanations for the disappointing results while acknowledging the possibility that these interventions simply "do not work."[34]

Is there a solution?

The ineffectiveness of interventions aimed at changing the public's dietary habits is indeed a complex issue that raises several questions: Why do obesity experts and diet gurus promote policies that don't work? Why don't these policies work? Finally, what might work instead? These are hard questions without simple answers.

Dietary habits are deeply ingrained and influenced by various factors such as culture, social norms, personal preferences, and accessibility to healthy foods. Changing these habits requires addressing multiple interconnected factors simultaneously, which can be challenging for interventions designed around a single approach or strategy.

Lack of sustained motivation and adherence to new dietary recommendations is a common issue. People may initially embrace changes but struggle to maintain them in the long term due to various factors including conflicting priorities, limited resources, and the influence of advertising and marketing for unhealthy foods.

The food environment's complexity also plays a significant role. The easy availability and affordability of processed and unhealthy foods, coupled with the pervasive marketing and advertising of such products, can undermine efforts to promote healthier choices.

It's been said that by regulating and monitoring the retail food environment, governments could help people help themselves by increasing access to affordable, nutritious foods.

Would this work? Can the government regulate the number and opening times of convenience stores? Would subsidies designed to lower the prices of healthy food increase their availability and accessibility to the people most at risk for obesity in the places where they shop? I have my doubts. Some countries have imposed serious restrictions on food marketing and advertising, particularly those targeting children. Such action can help reduce the influence of persuasive marketing techniques that often promote unhealthy choices. Some countries have banned junk food sales to children altogether. In the US, cities including Philadelphia, San Francisco, and Seattle levied a tax on sugary beverages. In 2021, a UNICEF-led consortium suggested prioritizing healthy options and even approved a "Right to Adequate Food" law to help transform the global food environment.[35]

Since there's a strong association between local retail food environments and obesity and related metabolic diseases, can we do more for the millions of US households that live more than a mile from a supermarket and don't have easy access to transportation? Can governments impose zoning and licensing regulations affecting the placement and density of food retail establishments? Would this help prevent an overconcentration of unhealthy food outlets in certain areas while increasing the availability of fresh produce and nutritious options? Would licensing requirements ensure that food establishments meet certain health and safety standards? Only time will tell, but these are Herculean tasks.

It's encouraging that public discourse about obesity and policymaking now reflects science. Policymakers and the public realize that obesity and related metabolic diseases are not just about people's food decisions. We now know that people are prone to over-consume unhealthy foods because our food environment exploits their vulnerabilities, undermining their ability to take responsibility for their food choices. But we need more research to understand which interventions will work best.

While regulating the retail environment isn't a panacea, under-standing how the food environment influences our weight can help policymakers identify ways to change the setting and, in turn, reduce the risk of obesity. And this heightened understanding may help address one of the obesity epidemic's more troubling trends: higher obesity rates among low-income and racial/ethnic minority groups. In these communities, traditional diet education campaigns seldom reach their intended targets, or, more often than not, people ignore them. So, we need a new paradigm.

Finally, we mustn't forget that managing the 24-hour food environment is just one piece of the puzzle. Only by tackling the complex system of influences that result in obesity can we reverse the epidemic.

Talley's Take: The Athlete Paradox

What's the first thing that comes to mind when you think of the world's greatest athletes?

Self-confidence, discipline, focus, poise under stress, fitness, and superior nutrition—these men and women are at the top of their game, striving for an edge over the competition. We hear so much about "marginal gains" in today's sports arena, it seems impossible that elite athletes and teams would leave any stone unturned in the quest for glory.

Indeed, daily training and recovery require a comprehensive

eating plan that matches competitive sports' physical and mental demands. We take for granted that the best athletes eat only the healthiest diet, relying on personal chefs or leading nutritionists to ensure they eat as clean as possible. A kale smoothie and a plate full of steamed salmon, vegetables, and sweet potato seem like the ideal meal for peak athletic performance.

Yet many pro athletes have terrible nutrition, and even the elite of the elite are susceptible to weight gain and the 24-hour food environment's many temptations. One leading NBA player was famous for subsisting on candy while winning three consecutive NBA Defensive Player of the Year Awards. A former Cy Young Award–winning pitcher set multiple MLB pitching records on a steady diet of Taco Bell. Early in her playing career, a legendary tennis player put on 20 pounds in two weeks by simply eating too much food.

For many high-performance athletes, oatmeal, veggies, and brown rice don't add up. And neither do the calories. A bowl of oatmeal with milk gives you just 150 calories, and a cup of tofu only boasts 175. But processed junk foods—candy bars, cookies, Pop-Tarts—provide far more energy-replenishing calories per gram.

I typically advise people to eat 2,000 calories or less daily for weight maintenance, depending on their activity level. However, elite athletes can burn 15 to 20 calories in a single minute. At the height of their training, typically when they're not competing, athletes work out for four to six hours daily, meaning they have to replenish between 4,000 to 6,000 calories.

I see the questions now. "Mr. Talley, if I work out every day, can I eat like these guys?" In fact, my client Martha, a marketing executive and amateur triathlete, asked me that very question recently.

The simple answer is you can eat whatever you want. However, unless you're an Olympic-level cross-country skier, a professional tennis player, or even a ballet dancer who spends hours a day perfecting their craft, you'll never burn off more calories than you consume. As I tell my clients, you can't outrun a lousy diet, even if your name is Usain Bolt.

This brings me to another point. Even if you could exercise away all the calories you consume, is it wise to eat this way?

One argument I heard about junk food comes down to the word "processed." These foods are already processed when we put them in our bodies. For a marathoner, a race-day staple of Twinkies, fruit snacks, and Gatorade means her body has one less thing to do to that food. It's an odd way to look at things, but she's saving energy.

Please don't misunderstand me. I don't think it's wise to eat this way, athlete or not, and let me explain why. It's not simply a calories-in, calories-out conversation for world-class athletes and you. You want to consume foods that improve your game, not detract from it.

Some clients have asked if intense physical activity can off-set the impact of a poor diet. The best available data show that it can't. In fact, we have substantial evidence demonstrating how nutrition positively and negatively impacts performance. While it seems that some athletes succeed no matter what they put into their bodies, high physical activity levels don't counteract a poor diet's detrimental effects. In particular, a poor diet can sig-nificantly impact an athlete's durability and performance. A bad diet may lack essential nutrients, leading to inadequate energy levels, impaired recovery, and increased susceptibility to injuries. Nutrient deficiencies can compromise muscle strength, endur-ance, and overall athletic performance.

Specifically, insufficient intake of carbohydrates, proteins, fats, vitamins, and minerals can hinder an athlete's ability to meet the physical demands of training and competition. Without proper nutrition, the body may struggle to repair and build muscle, main-tain optimal energy levels, and support overall health.

Additionally, an unhealthy diet can contribute to weight issues, which may negatively affect an athlete's agility, speed, and overall mobility. It can also increase the risk of chronic conditions such as cardiovascular disease and diabetes, further compromising an athlete's long-term durability.

A quality diet is essential both for professional and amateur athletes alike. You may have heard talk about the importance of essential micronutrients—inorganic and organic elements that exist as solids, and also organic compounds such as vitamins and minerals. These micronutrients form bioactive compounds, generally proteins. They are not direct sources of energy but facilitate energy production and utilization from carbohydrates, fats, and proteins; transport oxygen and carbon dioxide; regulate fluid balance; and protect against oxidative damage. Since our bodies don't produce most of them, we must get them through food. Now, for example, imagine a diet without a micronutrient like iron, which is found in spinach, beef, lentils, kidney beans, and pumpkin seeds, and helps blood transport oxygen to muscles. Your muscles would not have the strength and endurance to perform optimally.

Athletes, especially female athletes, need more iron than the general population. Iron deficiency affects up to 52 percent of female athletes. We all lose iron through sweat, skin, urine, the gastrointestinal (GI) tract, and for women, during menstruation.

A poor diet also slows recovery and increases soreness after intense workouts and competitions. Training induces controlled levels of damage in your muscles. Your body then rebuilds stronger muscles, leading to growth in muscle mass and increased need for proper nutrition.

Also, a poor diet may not supply sufficient antioxidants, particularly vitamin C, found in high amounts in broccoli, peppers, and citrus fruits, and vitamin E, abundant in olive oil, nuts, and seeds. Your body needs antioxidants to prevent exercise-induced cell damage.

Of course, unwanted weight gain is the biggest consequence of an unhealthy diet. Overeating, even among pro athletes, is the most prominent cause of weight gain. Mindless eating, frequent snacking, and making calorie-rich, nutrient-poor dietary choices all promote excessive calorie intake.

So, what are your options if you eat poorly but are trying to achieve peak performance and avoid unwanted pounds?

Many of my NBA and MLB clients, who eat after night games and frequently travel during their seasons, ask for guidance in how to avoid the bad food trap.

When traveling, I tell players to pack many healthy snacks. My favorite options include whole or dried fruit; nuts in pre-portioned bags; whole-grain pretzels, crackers, and breadsticks; trail mix; and snack bars made with whole grains, nuts, and fruit with little added sugars. Grass-fed beef jerky, turkey jerky, and salmon jerky, and unsalted nut mixes in pre-portioned bags also work well.

In some sports, teams will set up buffets for the players. I tell them to choose grilled, steamed, broiled, or baked items instead of fried or sautéed. Also, consider salads with lean protein and a vinaigrette-based dressing, oatmeal, and eggs on whole-grain bread.

Before they grab a plate, I tell them to walk around the buffet and decide which foods they'll choose and which they should avoid. Then, we ask them to fill half their plate with fruits and vegetables, one-quarter of lean protein, and one-quarter of whole grains such as quinoa or sweet potato.

Finally, drink enough water so you don't get dehydrated. Consuming water before and during meals increases satiety and reduces calorie intake.

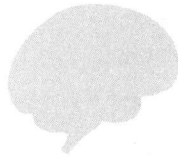

CHAPTER 9

Food Fight—The Body Politic's Messy Role in the Obesity Epidemic

There's little doubt that the standard American diet is causing widespread health problems. However, it's evident that politicians are not giving this problem the attention it deserves, despite the fact that obesity and related health issues are major contributors to our skyrocketing healthcare costs. The connection between what we eat and our well-being is often overlooked to the point where the government doesn't even keep track of annual spending on health-conscious initiatives, even in a country like the United States.

The government's lack of concern regarding the growing obesity crisis is almost comical. The cozy relationship many elected officials have with the food and beverage industry, and the government's overall disinterest in funding nutrition research, compounds this indifference. As a result, those who have the power to address obesity are doing little more than sitting on their hands.

Obesity presents a formidable political challenge. Regulatory interventions intended to tackle the obesity epidemic don't enjoy widespread support. Industry and powerful government interests routinely oppose helpful regulation. Our government, especially at the federal level, has opted for a "kid gloves" approach to dealing with obesity, including voluntary food labeling, fluffy social marketing campaigns, and school sports programs.

Little Appetite for Funding Nutrition Research

In recent years, while there has been some increase in funding for nutrition research, it's important to note that it has actually declined as a proportion of the overall National Institutes of Health (NIH) research budget. To illustrate, in 2018, the NIH allocated $1.8 billion for nutritional research, which represented slightly less than 5 percent of its total budget of $43 billion. Fast forward to 2022, when the NIH's total budget grew to $45 billion. Even with this increase, the NIH unveiled a plan in the same year to dedicate $170 million over five years to advance the relatively new field of precision nutrition. Despite this incremental rise in funding, it remains a modest allocation, especially when considering the pressing nature of the challenges we face in the realm of nutrition.[1]

For much of its history, nutrition research focused on identifying and preventing nutrient-deficiency diseases. However, today's diet crisis isn't one of deficiency; it's one of excess. Obesity costs taxpayers $147 billion to $210 billion annually in direct and indirect medical expenses. Similarly, diet-related diseases such as hypertension cost $131 billion, and diabetes, most of which is the type 2 variety, totals a whopping $237 billion.[2] Yet, despite what we know about the correlation between food intake and disease burden, no major lobbying force boosts nutrition research funding.

The lack of federal investment and interest in nutrition and its effect on human health has left an information void that the food industry has been happy to fill. However, food companies are not social service agencies. They're businesses, and like any money-making enterprise, they do everything possible to maximize sales and profits. So, it's no surprise that industry-supported nutrition studies are more about slick marketing than unbiased science.

Here's an example. In 2019, a major peer-reviewed study questioned the advice to eat less red and processed meat, pointing out the weak evidence backing such long-standing recommendations.[3] Conversely, a separate study published two years later found that the more red meat people consumed, the higher their risk of heart attack or stroke. After factoring in body weight, tobacco use, exercise, and specific eating habits, the risk rose, on average, by 22 percent for every daily serving of red meat.[4] These studies sparked the usual frenzy and yet another round of consumer confusion. It's easy to see why nutrition studies are the frequent butt of jokes. One day coffee is healthy; the next, it's not. Oh no! Even moderate alcohol consumption increases cancer risk. No wait, red wine is good for your heart. And hold on a minute—is cheese a healthy source of protein and calcium, or is it an inflammatory combination of salt and fat? Can someone please decide?

The research the federal government prioritizes rarely aligns with the prevalence of diseases. For example, in 2018, NIH funding for cancer, which despite considerable fanfare and attention affects less than 9 percent of the population, was $6.3 billion. Funding for obesity research, which affects about 42.4 percent of the country, was slightly more than $1 billion.[5]

Within the NIH, the fall of nutrition research goes beyond funding. There is no institute or center dedicated to the topic. There is no central leadership. Today, just a single office with a staff of four coordinates nutrition research.

The office isn't even on the NIH campus—symbolic of its lowly status. By contrast, a team of twenty-six people heads up the dietary supplements office, studying the effects of vitamins, minerals, and herbal remedies.

Even when former First Lady Michelle Obama waged a talked-about, single-woman war against childhood obesity, the federal government continued underfunding nutrition research. Without government support, the cost of dietary intervention studies skyrocketed. Today, most NIH grants cap at $500,000—a threshold that has not increased in a decade—and seldom come close to covering most clinical studies' exorbitant costs.[6] Without a significant public funding boost for nutrition research, there will be little progress against the obesity epidemic.

In 2016, the NIH created a nutrition task force to develop an agency-wide strategic plan to solicit broader research community input. A draft plan released in 2020 lays out some broad strokes and includes a lot of platitudes but does not mention funding. It only points out seven research gaps, such as the relationship between the diet and the gut microbiome and optimal nutrition during pregnancy and infancy to prevent chronic disease. The NIH plan still hasn't been finalized, and there's no timetable for its implementation. It feels like a futile exercise in virtue signaling.[7]

Nutrition Crisis: Can we recover from harm caused by decades of bad science?

I'm not breaking any new ground here by stating that nutrition science is in turmoil. Indeed, misinformation, disinformation, and fraud are rampant in nutrition science, partly because it's complicated.

A few years ago, several studies were published touting the health benefits of coffee. However, many of these studies were what we refer to as "observational studies," in which researchers followed coffee and non-coffee drinkers and monitored when and how they died. For decades, the nutrition field has relied on observational study data to get around problems inherent in clinical trials. Observational studies use self-reported data collected through surveys across populations to find associations with health outcomes. They are cheaper and less rigorous than randomized controlled trials (RCTs), even though RCTs are still the gold standard for studying the causal relationship between interventions and outcomes.

Observational studies are flawed because people often forget, exaggerate, or flat-out lie about what they eat, leading to conflicting headlines about everything from chocolate to red meat. However, most nutrition researchers contend these observational studies are essential, problems notwithstanding, because the findings can help develop dietary and health policies.

The problem arises when you search for differences between any two groups; you will find them. These studies didn't provide evidence of coffee's health benefits because they excluded many other variables that impact overall health. Regular coffee drinkers might have higher incomes, drink fewer sugary beverages, or lead more active lifestyles. Observational studies help identify trends but do not show cause and effect. To truly test whether coffee prevents a specific disease, researchers must conduct a randomized controlled trial.

In an RCT, researchers randomly assign volunteers to two groups, in this case one that will drink coffee and one that

continued

abstains. However, that's when the problems set in. First, you need compliance. Regular coffee drinkers won't give up their fixes without a fight, and people who don't drink coffee might be reluctant to start. And since you can't lock people in cages for weeks or months, there is no way of knowing whether they've done what you've asked. Even assuming the volunteers in the study play by the rules, there's still a possibility that some other significant difference exists between the two groups. Ultimately, these variables make it difficult to determine a definitive answer about coffee's health benefits.

So, while randomized controlled trials are the gold standard of nutrition research, they're not a silver bullet. They're long, detailed, and expensive. A large RCT across multiple sites can easily cost millions. And they sometimes raise ethical quandaries. If we had reason to suspect that coffee might be harmful, could we reasonably assign a group to drink coffee?

This discussion points out the poor state of nutrition science and the problems afflicting much of the research behind claims about the health benefits of particular foods and beverages.

No one would argue against diet as a cornerstone of a healthy lifestyle. Still, there's no way to know if coffee, turmeric, dark chocolate, or blueberries offer humans any tangible benefit.

And don't expect things to improve soon.

Siding with the Fattest Wallets: The Government's Sorry History with Food Policy

Did you know that Congress once declared pizza a vegetable?

Congress took this unusual action to protect this American

dietary staple from a nutritional overhaul of the public school lunch program. That was in 2011. A year earlier, the White House turned a blind eye and a deaf ear as Congress axed a plan by four federal agencies to reduce sugar, salt, and fat in food marketed to children.[8] Then, in November 2020, urged by the White House, the USDA reintroduced one percent chocolate milk in schools, cut whole-grain serving requirements by 50 percent, and gave school nutrition directors more time to meet weakened sodium (mostly from salt) reduction targets.[9]

Defeats such as these are commonplace because, at all levels of government, the food and beverage industries emerge victorious in every significant diet-related battle despite mounting scientific evidence of unhealthy food's effects.

It's an open secret that top food and beverage companies spend vast sums to strengthen and maintain their political influence in the fight to protect their billion-dollar bottom lines. And how much do they spend? According to Reuters, which analyzed decades-long lobbying records, the food and beverage industry more than doubled its spending inside the Beltway between 2019–2022.[10] In addition, an article on Food Dive, a site that monitors the food industry, reported that some of the biggest players, including Coca-Cola and PepsiCo, spent $38.2 million on lobbying in 2020 alone.[11] These companies dominate policymaking, vowing to make improvements while defeating government proposals to change the nation's eating habits.

Industry critics contend Washington has abandoned its effort to promote healthy eating, even after a high-profile push by current President Joe Biden, who organized the first-ever Conference on Hunger, Nutrition, and Health at the White House in September 2022. That no presidential administration—Democrat or Republican—has been able to change industry practices speaks to the food and beverage lobby's power and influence.

Limited Public Support for a Government Role in Reducing Obesity

Another issue thwarting a government-backed solution to the obesity epidemic stems from the public's ambivalence, as a Pew Research Center survey made clear. It's common knowledge that many politicians ignore their constituents' needs and concerns. However, nearly all want to win re-election, so they pay attention to opinion polls, which show that the public agrees on obesity's negative impact but not on the government's role in fixing it. While 69 percent of Americans see obesity as a severe public health problem, the public has mixed opinions about what the government should do about it. About 67 percent favor requiring chain restaurants to list calorie counts on menus. More than half (55 percent) of those surveyed favor banning TV ads of unhealthy foods during children's programming, but only a little more than one third (35 percent) support raising taxes on sugary soft drinks and unhealthy foods.[12]

This tepid support for government intervention in anti-obesity efforts doesn't surprise me. In the Pew survey, 22 percent said the government couldn't "do much," and 14 percent said their efforts wouldn't make a dent. Overall, 54 percent said the government should play little or no role.

Nowhere was this ambivalence about the government's role more obvious than in the great sin tax debate. Government officials always focus their anti-obesity efforts on the most obvious offender—food—notably, portion sizes and so-called sin taxes. While this might seem like a good idea, given that obesity foretells nearly sixty chronic and acute illnesses, attempts to pass portion-size and sin tax legislation rarely get off the ground.

Back in 2009, food and beverages companies were in a lather about a proposed penny-an-ounce tax on sugary drinks put forth by a Congress eager to raise money to pay for obesity-related health-care costs.[13] Predictably, the soda tax died in committee and, unlike Lazarus, still hasn't risen from the dead. In the intervening fourteen years, other proposed soda taxes have similarly fizzled. According to the American Beverage Association, twenty-four states and five cities have considered them.[14] In 2010, Washington state legislators approved a two-cent-a-can soda tax. Within one month, a trade group representing industry heavy hitters Coca-Cola, PepsiCo, and the Dr Pepper Snapple Group (now part of Keurig Dr Pepper) mounted a referendum campaign, spending $16 million to gather signatures and flood the airwaves. Eventually, the public voted 60 percent against the tax.

In 2014, New York State's highest court shut down New York City's infamous soda ban—the brainchild of former NYC Mayor Michael Bloomberg—which would've portion-capped sodas at 16 ounces.[15] In Los Angeles, the local government encouraged restaurants to offer smaller portion size options, healthier kids' menus, and free chilled water. Similarly, every US city, town, and municipality that suggested or implemented soda taxes to discourage sugary drink consumption has seen those efforts dropped or defeated.

The beverage industry spent $3.5 million to thwart Maine's 2008 soda tax attempt. Between 2009 and 2016, the American Beverage Association, Coca-Cola, and PepsiCo spent over $67 million to defeat soda taxes and warning labels in nineteen cities and states.[16] Soda tax proponents claimed victory following Philadelphia's implementation of a 1.5-cent-per-ounce tax that raised more than $200 million in 2017 when it first took effect. However, a Drexel University study found that Philly's soda tax had little impact on sweetened beverage consumption.[17] Indeed, Philly residents simply traveled outside the city limits to purchase soda. Meanwhile, decreased revenues forced several small groceries to shut their doors.

Passing the Buck

Food and beverage manufacturers and advertisers claim they aren't to blame for the country's staggering obesity rate. However, it seems they want absolution. They accept no responsibility, insisting they're part of the solution. Coca-Cola, PepsiCo, and Anheuser-Busch InBev, among many others, spend millions annually to ensure lawmakers and regulators hear their concerns. According to data from the Center for Responsive Politics, thirty food and beverage companies collectively spent $38.2 million on lobbying in 2020.[18] In contrast, the Center for Science in the Public Interest, a legitimate consumer advocacy group, spent about $40,000 lobbying in 2020 and roughly $320,000 total in 2022—which is what the food and beverage industry spends opposing stricter guidelines every few hours.[19, 20]

In 2022, Minnesota-based food manufacturing behemoth General Mills, one of the world's largest producers of sugary cereals and snacks, spent $730,000 on lobbying in the first half of 2022 alone—close to what it spent in all of 2021. The company also doubled its Washington lobbyist staff from three to six. And General Mills isn't the only Minnesota-based company currying favors from influential politicians. US Senator Amy Klobuchar (D-Minnesota) has a small stable of billionaire and billion-dollar corporate backers. Chief among them: Cargill, the Minneapolis-St. Paul–based agribusiness behemoth, and the United States' largest privately held company. Cargill has donated a small fortune in campaign contributions to Klobuchar over the course of her political career. And Cargill has a "hand in nearly every political office in Minnesota [and] all but one member of the state's congressional delegation received donations from Cargill in the 2018 election cycle," according to a Daily Beast exposé.[21]

Cargill is hardly the only company to target politicians. Since

2015, no company has doled out more lobbying cash than Coca-Cola, the world's largest nonalcoholic beverage company. In 2021, it spent $5.83 million on twenty-four lobbyists. While substantial, this dollar figure falls below the company's mean spending of $7.04 million over the past six years.[22]

Every Issue Is at Play

The food and beverage industry's lobbying efforts encompass many issues. As Marion Nestle, a former professor of nutrition, food studies, and public health at New York University, has pointed out, they'll lobby for and against anything that affects their business. Indeed, says Dr. Nestle, there isn't a single area of food or nutrition policy that escapes their reach. A big issue with lobbying is that it unfairly benefits deep-pocketed corporations whose wealth gets them special access to lawmakers, regulators, and other influential officials. Critics have long argued that lobbyists play an outsized role in influencing regulatory agency policy outcomes. Their connections create invaluable relationships and make it more likely that companies can mount a defense to quash proposed legislation that could potentially harm their bottom lines. They also fund seemingly benign nonprofits to work on their behalf. These nonprofits have very appealing names, such as the Center for Consumer Freedom, a Washington, DC-based nonprofit group founded in 1995 by lobbyist Rick Berman with a $600,000 Philip Morris contribution. It claims to fight against a "growing cabal of activists that has meddled in Americans' lives in recent years." This includes self-anointed food police, health campaigners, trial lawyers, personal-finance do-gooders, animal-rights misanthropes, and meddling bureaucrats, says Berman. The CCF claims food and restaurant companies fund their efforts, but the group's website doesn't list specific benefactors.[23]

Yet, the CCF spends a great deal of time lobbying politicians on behalf of its benefactors, which include the world's largest food and beverage companies. Berman even argued against a Mothers Against Drunk Driving initiative to lower the blood alcohol content (BAC) limit for drivers by claiming that the stricter limits would punish responsible social drinkers. Berman's true concern was more likely that lowering the BAC limit would hurt his client, the Miller Brewing Company. Berman's lobbying practices, and the catchy name of his nonprofit, are standard operating procedure in Washington, DC's corridors of power.

Borrowing from Tobacco's Playbook

Food and beverage companies claim they're making dramatic strides in self-regulation. However, they're moving at a snail's pace while trying to influence public opinion by using the same tactics tobacco companies use to defend their products.

How are the food and tobacco industries similar? Both industries challenge any links between their products and ill health. Both have rewritten product labels without making significant product changes. And both emphasize self-regulation, which is just a thinly veiled attempt to circumvent or preempt government standards. Both industries also market to kids, using what food and beverage watchdogs call "front groups," complete with those consumer-oriented names that hide their industry affiliations.

Semper Fries

In early 2023, the Biden administration announced more stringent nutrition guidelines for public school meals, which feed about 30 million students across 100,000 schools. The new rules, which will roll out gradually over the next few years, limit added sugars, including flavored milk. The rules also cut the allowable amounts of sodium and increase whole grain offerings.

The new guidelines are part of a larger USDA campaign to address the persistent and worsening problem of childhood obesity. By fall 2024, school offerings must include primarily whole-grain foods, with only occasional products containing refined grains such as those used in white pasta and white bread. The following years will see additional edicts like eliminating artificial sweeteners and lowering salt content.[24]

But not everyone is convinced this is the best approach.

On one side of the fence, the School Nutrition Association, another industry-supported front group, argues that "with no end in sight to supply chain and labor challenges, most school meal programs nationwide simply cannot meet these proposed nutrition mandates and exceed transitional standards," adding that the USDA ought to consider the potential negative impact of proposed rules on student meal participation.

This industry-supported association complained: "Students' tastes will not adjust to meals meeting stricter school nutrition standards when there are no mandatory nutrition standards for the commercial market or other federal nutrition programs . . . Since schools are the healthiest place Americans eat, a further drop in student meal participation would be contrary to goals of the Dietary Guidelines for Americans."[25]

Of the proposed changes to the school meal program, allowable salt has drawn the most attention. The American Heart Association argued that the sodium guidelines in the new standards fell way short of what they advocate. In contrast, the FDA initially praised the USDA's sodium reduction targets, noting that they reinforce the FDA's "signature efforts to improve our nation's nutrition" by establishing voluntary sodium reduction targets in recently released guidance.

But the USDA emphasized that the final rule, first published on February 7, 2022, outlining the transitional standards, was just that—transitional. The phased-in changes only cover 2023–2024. After that, the USDA wants long-term changes to align school nutrition standards with their updated Dietary Guidelines for Americans. The USDA said in a statement that it will "prioritize seeking input from schools, industry, and others to inform the process."[26] Notice what the USDA wrote. They will seek input from "industry and others to inform the process." So, they're telling you that the food and beverage industry will have a say in shaping school meal guidelines. Good luck with those sodium reductions.

A similar dust-up occurred after the Obama administration announced an overhaul to the school lunch program in 2011. Public health officials believed the most unhealthy items would drop off the government's $10.5 billion school lunch program when they announced the first menu overhaul in fifteen years.[27]

Then, like clockwork, Congress stepped in—at the behest of potato and pizza companies—to preserve French fries as a menu staple and to declare pizza, with its sugary tomato sauce, a vegetable.[28] Congressional meddling raises an important point: How can we count on politicians to act on our behalf when it's not in their interest to do so?

First Amendment Follies

For some time now, the food and beverage industry has argued that the First Amendment gives them the right to market foods any way they want. The Founding Fathers probably didn't envision food and beverage companies hijacking the First Amendment to defend their selling practices, but here we are. Many industry lawyers and lobbyists claim that since there's no hard proof that food marketing causes obesity, there's no legal basis for restricting ads. Food and beverage companies frequently align with advertisers to fight any regulations on food advertising.

Given all we know about the adverse health effects of certain foods, an interesting question comes to mind. Should food marketing and advertising enjoy the same First Amendment protections as newspaper columnists? Some public interest lawyers think the answer is no. One such person, Samantha Graff, an attorney with the National Policy & Legal Analysis Network to Prevent Childhood Obesity, co-authored two articles on the subject. She argues that the government can regulate food advertising because cognitive research shows it's inherently misleading. Graff and her colleagues assert, "Case law establishes that the First Amendment does not protect 'inherently misleading' commercial speech. In addition, cognitive research indicates that young children cannot effectively recognize the persuasive intent of advertising or apply the critical evaluation required to comprehend commercial messages. Given this combination, advertising to children younger than twelve should be considered beyond the scope of constitutional protection."[29]

The National Agricultural Law Center, which describes itself as a "nonpartisan, federally-funded source of objective, scholarly, and authoritative agricultural and food law research and information," states, "The First Amendment offers food companies some freedom to label their products as they wish and challenge compelled government disclosures. However, if the government can show a substantial benefit in prohibiting or requiring certain speech, and the government's action is reasonable, then a court may find that the regulation is constitutional."[30]

Since I'm writing a book about the global obesity epidemic, it would be easy to side with those who favor restrictions. After all, why even allow the advertising and marketing of unhealthy foods, which the American Psychological Association calls "unconscionable,"[31] given all we know about their effects on human health and contribution to the obesity epidemic?

Back in 2009, Congress passed a measure backed by Senator Tom Harkin (D-Iowa) and Senator Sam Brownback (R-Kansas) asking the Federal Trade Commission (FTC) and three other agencies—the CDC, the USDA, and the FDA—to draft voluntary nutrition standards for children's food marketing. The two senators' motivation came from two studies showing that children develop lifelong preferences from watching ads that target them with saltier, sweeter foods than adults.[32]

By the time the draft guidelines were finally published two years later—with praise from health groups—industry interests had already mobilized, claiming the low sugar and salt suggestions shocked them. Food companies, fearing the senators' recommendations could lead to new requirements and derail their food marketing efforts, quickly took action by creating another front group with a catchy name: the Sensible Food Policy Coalition (SFPC). The group funded a report claiming that the proposed restrictions would kill 75,000 jobs and cost food companies $28.6 billion in lost revenue— estimates based on the supposition that the guidelines would slash one in five food ads.[33]

Government officials and public health advocates countered, arguing that the food and beverage industries had five years to improve their products. Food industry supporters openly fretted that the voluntary food guidelines would become mandatory. Almost immediately, the industry-backed SFPC's report was widely circulated in corridors of power. It was signed by about two hundred members of Congress from both parties.[34]

One signatory, Senator Dick Durbin, is from Illinois, home to Kraft-Heinz, the country's fifth-largest food company. Kraft-Heinz's political action committee (PAC) has contributed thousands of dollars to Durbin's campaign committee since 2007.[35] Kraft-Heinz also employs thousands of Illinois residents and contributes billions annually in tax revenues. In time, the guidelines died on the vine. As one advocacy group policy director said, "We just got beat. Money wins."[36]

Toxic Corruption: How Chemical Companies Shape Policy and Obesity

Given all we know about the effects of toxic chemicals on human health, you'd think Washington would step in to save the day. Think again!

Turn back the clock to 1976, when Congress took a bold step to keep Americans safe from dangerous chemicals by passing the Toxic Substances Control Act (TSCA).[37] Think about that. Our nation's primary defense against environmental toxins comes from an era when Gerald Ford was the president, the Cold War was still raging, and the disco era was in full swing. In the intervening forty-six years, we've fallen off the proverbial cliff. Of the 82,000 chemicals registered for commercial use since the TSCA first went into effect, just 200 have undergone health and safety testing by the EPA, and new safety rules have been created for just five of them, according to a *National Geographic* report.[38] Scientists believe that in 2017 alone, exposure to just a fraction of over 100,000 commonly used chemicals contributed to 1.3 million premature deaths.[39]

Even a bill passed by the Senate in 2016, the Frank R. Lautenberg Chemical Safety for the 21st Century Act—designed to update the TSCA—contained serious loopholes that raised concerns among public health and safety advocates. And no surprise, the chemical industry's fingerprints—and checkbooks—are all over it.

The Loopholes

The Senate requires the EPA to review at least twenty chemicals simultaneously, each with a seven-year deadline. The industry had five years to comply. That's twelve years before we could make any meaningful change to chemical exposures we know are detrimental to human health. In addition, the new law required the EPA to test tens of thousands of unregulated chemicals currently on the market. While that seems like a great thing, what's gone almost unnoticed is that roughly 2,000 new chemicals are introduced every year, according to the United States Department of Health and Human Services' National Toxicology Program.[40] This quagmire puts the EPA in the unenviable position of being the proverbial Dutch boy trying to plug a small crack in a dam. Unfortunately, there are multiple holes in the EPA's dam, and another leak springs every time one gets filled. At this pace, the EPA would never finish its review and is effectively enjoined from acting against endocrine-disrupting toxic chemicals for years.

Many states have stepped in to protect their communities from toxic chemicals. And they've done a pretty good job. In 2022, Maine pushed for lower limits on toxic chemicals in drinking water. This addressed PFAS compounds. The state also implemented strict safety standards on PBDEs (used as fire retardants) and BPA. These state-level reforms prompted national changes, leading major toymaker Hasbro to remove BPA from its products. Senator Lautenberg's proposed bill doesn't undo existing state laws as the one in Maine does, but it would prevent states from enacting future reforms.

The advocates of the Lautenberg proposal claim states aren't permanently banned from acting on these chemicals. However, they're in limbo because EPA reviews take time—sometimes decades. As investigative reporter Sharon Lerner observed, "The EPA has been investigating the safety of some of the flame retardants that the Washington state bill would ban for over 25 years. And the agency has spent at least 30 years looking at the safety of methylene chloride, which is still widely available in hardware stores though its fumes have been killing people since at least the 1940s."[41]

And that's just one escape hatch in the Senate bill. Another loophole threw a monkey wrench into the EPA's plan to prevent foreign products containing dangerous chemicals from being imported into the United States. This move made it even easier for toxic toys, furniture, and other consumer products to appear in American stores and homes.

Yet another loophole pushed the EPA to designate many chemicals as "low priority" without a complete evaluation. And, perhaps most troublingly, neither the Senate nor House version of the bill requires companies to prove new chemicals are safe from a health perspective before bringing them to market.[42]

How did all these loopholes make it into the final Senate bill? That's easy. Like their food and beverage counterparts, the chemical industry spent tons of money influencing the legislation. The US chemical industry is a monster, responsible for $5.2 trillion in business activity—or approximately a quarter of our GDP—and about 4.1 million jobs.[43] With so much money at stake, is it any wonder that the pending TSCA updates had the blessings of two leading chemical industry lobbyists, the American Chemistry Council and the American Petroleum Institute? When Senators David Vitter and Frank Lautenberg introduced a TSCA reform bill on May 22, 2013, interest groups supporting the legislation directed more than

$54 million in political contributions to US senators, outspending an opposing coalition of consumer rights and public health advocacy groups by an eight-to-one margin. The aforementioned American Chemistry Council likely wrote entire portions of the Senate legislation, say many experts.[44]

Two former senators, Tom Udall (a New Mexico Democrat and now the US ambassador to New Zealand) and David Vitter (a Louisiana Republican), made up the bipartisan team that helped push the legislation through the Senate while they were still seated. They also benefited from the chemical industry's largesse. The chemical industry gave then-Senator Udall tens of thousands of dollars and ran TV ads on his behalf. Former Senator Vitter also attracted significant donations from the chemical industry, which gave generously to his campaign and a super PAC supporting his failed bid for Louisiana governor.[45]

Playing by Their Own Rules

As usual, industries willing to spend big on political contributions and lobbying get to write their own rules. As the federal government and Congress have increased efforts over the last few years to regulate per- and polyfluoroalkyl substances (PFAS), major chemical manufacturers have ramped up their political lobbying and donation campaigns. The chemical industry spent almost $66 million lobbying Congress in 2022, according to campaign finance records published on OpenSecrets.org.[46] The seven largest PFAS producers and their trade groups spent at least $61 million in 2019 and 2020, largely to successfully lobby Congress against PFAS legislation and rules, according to *The Guardian*.[47]

The chemical industry marshaled its efforts to defeat many proposals compelling companies to pay for cleaning up widespread

PFAS pollution. Lobbying records show PFAS manufacturers like Chemours, 3M, DuPont, Daikin, Arkema, Solvay, and the American Chemistry Council trade group dispatched lobbyists to Congress, where they donated to key congressional lawmakers debating the bill.[48] Chemical industry lobbyists use tactics similar to tobacco and oil lobbies, aiming to "create a cloud of doubt" over clear science showing PFAS' health threat. The strategy has successfully delayed new regulations. Such lobby spending by chemical industry players will remain high for the foreseeable future because the EPA under President Joe Biden has already proposed PFAS restrictions the chemical industry opposes.[49] As a result, any meaningful PFAS legislation will probably die on the vine in Congress.

My Take

We live in a time when hundreds of millions of people lack adequate food, but just as many, if not more, are obese to the point of increased risk for diet-related chronic diseases. Food companies aren't stupid: they're well aware of the economic implications of reversing the obesity epidemic, as are government agencies. As Marion Nestle points out, "Economists at the US Department of Agriculture (USDA) calculate that 'large adjustments' would occur in the agriculture and processed food industries if people ate more healthfully."[50] In other words, food and beverage companies would lose big bucks.

The prospect of billions of lost revenue is one reason food producers contribute generously to political campaigns and why federal agencies have failed to take the obvious first step: a government-sponsored national obesity-prevention campaign. Such a campaign would have to address dietary aspects, including messages to eat less and (less controversially) move more. Since no federal health agency has stepped in to take the lead on dietary issues, the USDA is left in charge of national nutrition policy, akin to placing a fox in charge of guarding the henhouse. Remember, the USDA primarily promotes US agricultural products, hence it is in their interest for people to "eat more." Yet, it also issues advice about diet and health—an apparent conflict, accounting for the ambiguity of federal dietary guidelines.

Given that promoting healthy eating may not align with the interests of the food industry, and given that government agencies are potentially influenced, addressing the obesity epidemic in the US presents a significant challenge. The sheer magnitude and extent of this epidemic necessitates a more deliberate and comprehensive approach to understanding obesity and the impact of our dietary choices. To tackle this issue effectively, we should reconsider campaign contribution and lobbying regulations and advocate for the establishment of a government-sponsored agency, independent of industry and congressional influence, with a clear mandate for overseeing matters related to food, nutrition, and health. Essentially, we require an external entity to oversee these critical areas.

Recognizing these barriers to regulation and taking proactive measures to surmount them is essential for future endeavors to succeed at preventing obesity.

Both sides of the political aisle must acknowledge that the food industry isn't the American public's friend and only acts in its own self-interest, even if that means impeding progress on government-sanctioned obesity prevention policies. Getting smarter about these issues is the first step in turning things around. Without that, even a joint public-private approach to dealing with the obesity epidemic is bound to fail.

Talley's Take: Kyle's Quandary— Solving a Teen's Sudden Weight Gain

"I don't get it. We eat well at home. We keep junk food out of the house. He's active and plays two varsity sports. Can you tell me why my kid is gaining so much weight?"

My client Harry, a famed sports and entertainment attorney, is clearly frustrated. In the past year, his son, Kyle, a high school sophomore, had put on 65 pounds.

"How can a sixteen-year-old, two-sport athlete put on that much weight?" he asked rhetorically.

"Have you been to the doctor?" I responded.

"Of course, we took him to the pediatrician, endocrinologist, and a nutritionist. They ran a dozen tests, and everything was fine. There's nothing abnormal except the weight spike."

After listening to Harry, who'd dropped 50 pounds in the last eighteen months, I told him the best thing to do was to bring Kyle in. A week later, Kyle was sitting in my office. It was obvious he'd put on a lot of weight, mostly around his waist and thighs.

"Kyle, you're here because your dad is concerned about your weight. I'm interested in hearing your thoughts."

Kyle paused for a moment before answering. "For sure, I've gained a few pounds, but I'm not sure why. I don't think I'm doing anything different."

As we started talking, Kyle casually mentioned that he'd recently switched schools, leaving the small private school he'd attended since kindergarten for a much larger public high school, which along with stellar academics, happened to have one the state's best lacrosse teams. Kyle was a top lacrosse player and had been named to the list of the country's "25 High School Boys' Lacrosse Players to Watch." He even dreamed of playing lacrosse at his dad's alma mater, Yale, on the country's eleventh-ranked team.

Kyle's athletic prowess (he also played linebacker on the school's varsity football team and trained six days a week) made his weight gain even more shocking.

So, I started probing.

"What do you eat on a typical day?" I asked.

"I don't know. My mom makes me breakfast at home. Usually eggs and toast. Then I have something at school with my friends before class."

"What do you have before class?"

"I don't know. A bag of Doritos or pretzels, maybe some cupcakes or a candy bar."

"Do you do this every day?"

"Sure. Everyone does," he said.

"Where do you get this food?"

"From the vending machines. There are five of them at school," he said.

Now, Kyle's weight gain made sense. After reviewing what Kyle typically ate from the school vending machines, I estimated that he was getting an extra 10,000 calories a week. Local school boards have to accept whatever the federal government sends to them. The relationship between local school boards and the federal government in the realm of school lunch programs is governed by a combination of funding, nutritional guidelines, and the broader goal of promoting students' health and well-being. However, it's a whole different ball game when school boards are paid off by junk food distributors to fill school machines with their products. Vending machines may contribute to childhood obesity because of the food they contain.

Once I identified the source of Kyle's weight gain, fixing the problem got much easier. Since Kyle was training several hours a day, he was always hungry and thirsty. I started out by recommending he carry a thermos or water bottle he could refill throughout the day. Water is a natural appetite suppressant. When the stomach senses that it is full, it sends signals to the brain to stop eating. Water can help to take up space in the stomach, leading to a feeling of fullness and reducing hunger.

I also suggested to Kyle, and his dad, that he pack his own healthy snacks. He could make and bring a sandwich, cut up vegetables, chips and cheese, a salad, fruit, granola bars—the options were endless. I also told Kyle that whatever he chose, each snack should contain protein and fiber to help him feel full faster and longer. When Kyle told me he would feel ridiculous bringing food to school, I told him to think back to when he was little and his mom packed him a lunch and snack every day. "You would be mad if she forgot, so why should you?" I said.

Finally, I reminded Kyle to never go hungry because that's when he would certainly resort to an unhealthy option. If you're starving, you're more apt to overeat.

Kyle's story should remind us of the food industry's powerful impact on young people. These advertisements often utilize colorful packaging, animated characters, and catchy slogans to make unhealthy food products more attractive to the younger demographic. Constant exposure to such messaging can contribute to the development of poor eating habits, leading to an increased consumption of processed and sugary foods, which in turn is linked to a higher risk of obesity and other health issues.

As Dr. Lonky points out in this chapter, one significant challenge in addressing this issue is the lack of sufficient regulation around advertising potentially harmful foods to young audiences. While some governments have implemented restrictions on advertising certain foods during children's programming, there is often a gap in regulations for online platforms, social media, and other non-traditional advertising channels. Additionally, the definition of "unhealthy" foods and the criteria for regulating them vary across regions, making it challenging to establish consistent guidelines. The absence of comprehensive regulations allows for the continuous bombardment of persuasive messages promoting unhealthy food choices to young people, contributing to a concerning public health issue that demands attention and action.

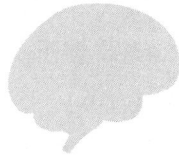

CHAPTER 10

Fat Habits—The Little Understood Role of Human Behavior on Obesity

Mary's Story

My patient Mary has been a picture of good health for most of her life. She exercises regularly, eats a balanced diet, manages stress, and enjoys healthy personal and professional relationships. So, Mary couldn't understand why she was gaining weight. She saw her internist and OBGYN, and after extensive testing, they ruled out any underlying medical conditions contributing to her recent and rapid weight gain, including thyroid deficiency and polycystic ovary syndrome (PCOS).

However, Mary had put on enough weight that her BMI was hovering around 30, putting her squarely in the mildly obese category. Soon after, she developed exertional dyspnea and obstructive sleep apnea syndrome (OSAS). Mary came to see me at her internist's recommendation to deal with her respiratory complaints. Taking steps to relieve Mary's dyspnea and OSAS was important. However, I wanted to understand why Mary had put on so much weight.

As we talked, Mary mentioned that her mother had died during the early stages of the COVID pandemic. Like millions of Americans, Mary had turned to food to cope with both pandemic-related stress and the grief brought on by her mother's unexpected passing. The years of careful meal planning and prepping on which Mary prided herself gave way to sugary cereal, baked goods, processed foods, and food delivery services. Mary's gym also shuttered its doors for fifteen long months. The abrupt disruption of Mary's routines coupled with the stress and anxiety of losing her mother kept these unhealthy behaviors in place. For example, Mary got into the unconscious habit of snacking whenever an uncomfortable feeling surfaced. She'd munch on a bag of chips while working, watching TV, or talking on the phone. Before long, Mary would reach into the bag only to find it empty. "I don't understand how I ate that many chips," she confided.

I reminded Mary not to feel bad because this phenomenon happens to more people than you think. The mindless or emotional eating concept stems from psychological behaviors stimulated by a distracted brain and habitual behavioral repetition. Sometimes eating has nothing to do with food.

Mindless eating is the idea that our unconscious decisions about food can profoundly affect our diet and weight. In contrast to mindful eating, which promotes behaviors such as slow eating without distraction and an appreciation of your food's smell and texture, mindless eating is distracted eating.[1] It's a disconnection from the way we experience food and its impact on our bodies. A clear illustration of this is eating when you're not actually hungry. Considering that it can take your brain up to twenty minutes to register fullness, it's evident how thoughtless eating habits can contribute to weight gain. Another example of this is eating too rapidly, which can not only leave you physically uncomfortable but also mentally stressed, often accompanied by a form of guilt for consuming more food than you intended.[2]

Human Behavior: Obesity's Missing Link

Of all the factors contributing to the obesity epidemic, behavior might be the most underappreciated and least understood. Indeed, looking at all the obesity epidemic's antecedents, the experts devote comparatively little attention to human behavior's influence on our weight. Suppose, for example, energy expenditure was obesity's leading cause. In that case, an obvious solution would be eating less and exercising more. However, millions of people have walked that path, and it just hasn't worked.

Here's the fundamental problem with the energy balance model, not to mention most weight-loss programs. Solutions to obesity's rapid rise typically rest on three false assumptions:

1. Most people can eat moderately, i.e., enjoy all foods in moderation.

2. Individual willpower is enough to lose weight and sustain weight loss.

3. Eating behavior is a rational process, controllable with logic and reason.

After nearly five decades of medical practice and research, I can confidently say these assumptions have no bearing on real-world eating behavior. They also explain why lasting weight loss is a Sisyphean task for most people.

We've seen dramatic changes to the modern food environment in the last few years. Most Americans get their calories from inexpensive, high-calorie, and highly refined carbohydrates. This increased availability has been coupled with documented increases in portion size and the caloric density of many common foods, contributing to a 24 percent rise over consumption levels in 1961, when the average was just 2,880 calories.[3]

I don't want to dismiss nutrition science's role in educating the public about the relationship between diet and health. However, few people adhere to guidelines set forth by public health officials, physicians, nutritionists, and other self-styled experts despite relative scientific consensus on the constituents of a healthful diet. The demand for high-calorie on-the-go snacks, fast foods, and ready-made meals has never been higher.[4] Don't believe it? Try visiting your local Chick-fil-A or Shake Shack around dinner time. There's no point in denying this reality. Just as we know it's better to live within our means and avoid overspending, most people know how they should behave around food. But how do they really behave? Well, they *misbehave*. And there's no sign of a slowdown, despite research showing that the typical dieter makes four or five weight-loss attempts annually (meaning the typical dieter is failing four or five times annually).[5]

Efforts to treat, reverse, and prevent obesity have focused on enhancing public awareness via government and non-governmental organization (NGO) messaging and providing information on the healthiest diet and the benefits of regular physical activity. This focus exists across all government-sanctioned programs, popular industry diets such as Weight Watchers, and dozens of diet books. Calorie restriction—through portion control or excluding/demonizing entire food groups—is a hallmark of most weight-loss programs. As I mentioned, this effort rests on a faulty assumption—that human eating behavior is rational, conscious, and knowledge-based. This assumption is simply *wrong*.

How do we know this? Just look at the success and failure rates of most weight programs. They help people lose small amounts of weight over a limited time period. That's why we call it "yo-yo dieting." However, even the most intensive diet cannot help people keep the weight off. In reality, most dieters regain everything they lose and then some within five years.[6] Obesity research doesn't reflect this because it rarely follows people for more than eighteen months, a problem affecting many weight-loss studies.

Most weight-loss programs are inadequate, offering what I'd charitably describe as an incomplete approach to lasting weight loss. As an example, in the Weight Watchers system, food is assigned a number of points, and a breadstick is only worth one point, whereas a piece of chocolate cake comes in at four points. To the casual observer, choosing the low-calorie breadstick over the high-calorie cake seems like a simple decision. The problem is that the breadstick might trigger cravings in someone who overeats bread products or baked goods. I know it seems strange, but that simple breadstick or roll could reactivate a habit pattern that leads a susceptible person to over-consume baked goods. In no time, that 20-calorie breadstick could become thousands of added calories.

Here's an example from my life. My wife has a weakness for toffee; Heath bars are her Achilles' heel. While they make miniature versions, or you can easily break off a piece of the larger size bar, she will keep eating them. She can't stop at one or two bites. The toffee triggers a reaction that does not involve taste or hunger. It's a compulsion, and having a little of a compulsion is hard. Her solution: We don't keep toffee in our house. After all, you can't eat what isn't there. Ice cream is my food weakness. I am not even aware of how much I am eating. Ironically, I stop craving it after a single scoop but keep going.

Much of the blame for our weight-loss failures rests with gurus who, in my view, overemphasize the importance of human agency, moderation, willpower, and rational decision-making. These broad assumptions about human behavior help fuel the obesity epidemic. I want to be clear: I don't believe there's any possibility of reversing the obesity epidemic without a commitment to lasting behavioral change.[7] Therefore, I'm wary of anyone who thinks we can address obesity strictly from a nutritional point of view.

Why We Fail

Have you ever heard the expression, "Everything in moderation"? It's a ubiquitous bit of healthy eating advice offered by lifestyle gurus, celebrities, and even nutritionists. It also dates back thousands of years to the Greek poet Hesiod, who famously opined, "Moderation is best in all things." However, just because a saying has persisted over time doesn't mean it's correct, helpful, or valuable. As the inimitable nineteenth-century playwright Oscar Wilde—a keen observer of human nature—once said, "Everything in moderation, including moderation." Wilde's take on this ancient maxim reveals its inherent folly. Moderation is for whatever you want, when you want it. Or, as cardiologist and Tufts University professor of nutrition science Dariush Mozaffarian told the *New York Times*, "The notion that it's OK to eat everything in moderation is just an excuse to eat whatever you want."[8]

While "all foods in moderation" seems like sensible advice for people with weight problems, the expression is problematic because "moderation" is subjective. Indeed, of the many false assumptions made and promoted about human eating behavior, none have done as much damage as the premise that people can eat moderately. Unfortunately, there's scant evidence suggesting that this is true. More than likely, the opposite is true. Think about it: How many heavy people do you know who eat moderately? Without firm guidelines and clear boundaries, a "moderate" serving of any food becomes an elastic concept that depends on a person's perception, upbringing, and psychological makeup.

Not only is "all foods in moderation" meaningless, but it probably harms people trying to maintain or lose weight, according to the University of Georgia and Duke University researchers. These researchers conducted a study involving 504 in-person participants and online respondents. They found that most people think the concept of "moderation" is more extensive than the recommended amounts a person should eat.[9]

Moderation doesn't work for most people because human behavior leans toward immediate gratification and excess, especially when engaging in pleasurable activities such as eating. The interaction between human behavior and eating patterns/habits is far more critical than any discussion about the fat, calories, and grams of sugar in a doughnut or chocolate chip cookie. I have a patient who grew up hearing from her mother that in polite society people always leave some food on their plates. While that might seem like a great idea, it ignores an obvious reality about human behavior: People, especially those with weight problems, are finishers. Most people clean their plates, regardless of portion size. Telling them to leave some food on their plate is torture, particularly if they're enjoying a celebratory meal.

The idea of finishing everything on your plate also has cultural and historical backing. During World Wars I and II, governments encouraged citizens to avoid wasting food as part of the war efforts. Rationing was implemented, and governments urged citizens to be mindful of their food consumption to support the troops and ensure everyone had enough to eat. The Clean Plate Club idea gained popularity during these times, as finishing one's plate was seen as a patriotic act and a way to contribute to the war effort.

And even before that, during the Great Depression in the 1930s, which led to widespread economic struggles, conserving resources, including food, became crucial. The Clean Plate Club concept was reinforced during this period to minimize food waste. In the mid-twentieth century, with an increasing focus on nutrition and health, the Clean Plate Club was also promoted to ensure that individuals received adequate nutrients. Parents often encouraged their children to finish their plates to ensure they were getting the necessary vitamins and minerals.

In time, the Clean Plate Club concept became ingrained in American culture and was often passed down through generations as a well-intentioned practice. It was commonly associated with values of discipline, gratitude, and thriftiness.

Here's another reality about human behavior that the experts frequently ignore: We're programmed to over-consume. And the ingredients in many food products—fat, sugar, and salt—fuel this tendency, destroying our evolutionary ability to achieve and maintain metabolic homeostasis and control our weight. This ingredient combo activates the brain's reward system—the mesolimbic dopamine system—reinforcing reward behaviors.[10] Our inclination toward immediate gratification (be it drugs, alcohol, shopping, or highly palatable food), and the overlapping and redundant neural reward mechanisms that drive and reinforce such pleasure-driven behavior, make moderation almost impossible. Therefore, the select few who succeed at weight control exclude certain foods, particularly those they overeat, instead of trying to cut a deal with them. Don't negotiate with a cupcake, peanuts, or any food you have a history of overeating. You'll lose every time.

Weighing In on Willpower

"You want fries with that?"

You would be in good company if you answered "yes" to that question. However, a more pressing question is *why* you answered "yes." Most French fries are high in calories and unhealthy fat; unless we're talking about sweet potato fries, they're not nutrient-dense. So, why would you eat them? What's wrong with you? Honestly, you're probably fine. As one of my colleagues famously said, "You don't have to be crazy to be crazy about a cookie." And here's a shocker: you might be in for one hell of a surprise if you think the answer to the fries question has anything to do with willpower or self-control.

Time after time, I've observed that the willpower muscle doesn't translate to eating behavior. Take the example of my patient Henry, one of Los Angeles' most successful real estate developers. He's been married to the same woman for thirty-two years, and they have three beautiful kids and a grandchild on the way. He's successful in every area except one: He can't control himself around baked goods, especially bread products. He will often sit at a restaurant and polish off a bread basket before dinner. Henry's struggles with baked goods remind me that millions of people with weight problems also enjoy great personal and professional success and accomplish many things that require dedication, perseverance, and self-control. Their failures in this one particular area point out something amiss in our complex relationship with food.

While evidence suggests that willpower is excellent for short-term behavior change, e.g., dieting to slim down from a size 8 to a size 6, it's of little benefit for lasting weight loss.[11] I have another patient, Joey, who, after much prodding, added exercise to his daily regimen. Joe followed a strict diet for months and made some progress but then plateaued. And to his credit, he stuck with a weightlifting and cardiovascular exercise program five to six days a week. But that's when the problems kicked in. On a recent visit to my office, Joey was noticeably heavier. He confided that he'd gained 10 pounds in just three weeks. I asked about his daily diet and exercise regimen. Was he sticking with the program? Within a few minutes, it was obvious why he was packing on the pounds. Joey had developed a post-workout routine that looked something like this: After a long workday, followed by his daily workout, he'd sit on the couch and veg out for hours, doing what he called "sports and chill," which meant watching his favorite teams while keeping company with a quart of ice cream or bag of chips. Even though he knew eating ice cream or chips and sitting for a long time were terrible ideas, he convinced himself that this nightly downtime was a well-deserved reward for all his hard work.

Psychological researchers have a name for this phenomenon: *ego depletion*. The theory is that willpower is connected to a limited reserve of mental energy, and once that energy runs out, our self-control goes out the window.[12] This theory would seem to explain Joey's after-work indulgences perfectly.

When it comes to weight management, willpower's reality aligns with short-term dieting success. It's a fragile foundation for weight control and is easily compromised.

To me, willpower is like arm wrestling against a much larger opponent. You can probably hang in for a bit, but your muscles will eventually fatigue, and your arm will give way. In a recent study, researchers found that people who used willpower to resist cookies and candy were more likely to throw in the towel in a follow-up puzzle task than those who hadn't used willpower. The authors said that exercising willpower had taxed participants' resources to such a degree that they couldn't complete an unrelated task.[13]

There's a correlation here with our 24-hour food environment, where the constant exposure to and availability of highly palatable food requires an iron will and unwavering self-control. In many areas of human engagement, willpower is incompatible with human behavior. As biological, psychological, and environmental cues converge, the likelihood increases that we'll do something not in our best interests. For an obese person, that could mean eating well beyond their nutritional or hunger needs.

Innate biological and evolutionary mechanisms that promote food consumption further tax willpower. Think about it. Dieting is all about reducing calories. However, when we lower food intake, hormonal and metabolic shifts create an intense desire and craving for food. For example, neuropeptide-Y, a neurotransmitter that stimulates food intake and increases the motivation to eat and delays satiety, will wreck any attempt at calorie restriction.[14] Other studies suggest that weight loss unfavorably changes hormones linked to appetite regulation, including leptin, insulin, neuropeptide-Y, and ghrelin. These changes subsequently increase hunger and food drive. This effect is so powerful that the appetite-promoting pattern continues for one year after weight loss and never reverts to pre-weight-loss levels![15, 16]

Food manufacturers also play a role here. Business entities and other critical contributors to our food environment rely on continued product consumption to maintain profitability. They are adept at eroding our willpower. Increasing product consumption is the food industry's goal and focus, not weight loss or healthy eating. Never forget that.

Perhaps the clearest example of industry-driven consumption was in the 1980s when Frito-Lay released an advertising campaign featuring the tagline "Bet you can't eat just one." Frito-Lay's slogan wasn't just a marketing bonanza—it also revealed an essential truth about human behavior. For millions, the momentary pleasure of a salty, crunchy chip somehow outweighs the future promise of fitting into a pair of skinny designer jeans or the desire to live a healthier life. To give up future good health for a few seconds of ecstasy might seem irrational, but it's also entirely predictable. Human eating behavior is seldom rational. Behavioral biases, including a greater emphasis on immediate or present gratification rather than delayed gratification, are part of the human condition.

Why do today what you can put off till tomorrow?

Procrastination is the best-known behavioral bias. Why do people spend hours scrolling through Instagram or watching TikTok videos instead of finishing an assignment or work project? I can tell you laziness isn't driving this behavior. It's not simply wanting to avoid the day's task or chore but more about human wiring. We're biased toward the present, meaning we prefer short-term rewards that provide instant gratification.

Intuitively, we understand that the benefit of losing weight far outweighs the momentary pleasure of a piece of chocolate cake. But we're programmed to hunt for that immediate dopamine hit. Similarly, we'll opt for a handful of crunchy, salty chips today while promising to start dieting tomorrow. But in the blink of an eye, tomorrow becomes today, and we have another handful of chips and put off the diet for another day.

It's no mystery why we're biased toward the present. Uncertainty governs human existence. Even in the relative safety and comfort of modern society, our lives can end without notice. Why put off something pleasurable until tomorrow or next week when there might not be a tomorrow or next week? Ironically, multiple studies show delayed gratification's benefits. Years ago, a psychologist, Walter Mischel, conducted his famous marshmallow test to determine whether children can delay gratification. Dr. Mischel asked the children to choose a marshmallow now or wait fifteen to twenty minutes to get two. This experiment, however, did not end there. After a few years, these same children who delayed gratification were more successful overall, shedding light on how small decisions can become a habit.[17]

Since our minds view the future as uncertain, they want to make decisions that impact the present, even if they're not beneficial. Behavioral economists use *present bias* when discussing time inconsistency and discounting. Time inconsistency means we exhibit a "present bias," whereby we ascribe more "value" to the present than the future. For instance, you decide to join a gym next month. However, when the next month arrives, you're more likely to postpone it to the following month, and so on.

Since it is wired into our system to focus on the present while discounting future consequences, present bias manifests in many actions. How else to explain why we eat poorly and gain weight? A pound here or there doesn't seem like a clear and present danger. However, we should understand that our brains aren't always thinking about what's best for us, resulting in impulsive decision-making that might lead to future disasters. Remember the quote from *Forbes* columnist Bruce Y. Lee about obesity being a "catastrophe in slow motion"? We don't notice obesity because it happens slowly, often over many years. We must be more aware of how our brains trick us, and maybe not always trust that "inner voice."

Early on, I learned from behavioral economics that unseen and seldom discussed forces, not rational decision-making, drive our most important decisions. Indeed, not only do we make obvious mistakes, but we repeat the same mistakes again and again. We are, in the words of Duke University psychologist and behavioral economist Daniel Ariely, "predictably irrational." As Dr. Ariely points out in his *New*

York Times bestseller, *Predictably Irrational,* when it comes to making important decisions, we habitually delude ourselves into thinking we're making smart, rational choices. From drinking coffee and losing weight, to buying a car and choosing a romantic partner, we consistently overpay, underestimate, and procrastinate. Yet, these misguided behaviors are neither random nor senseless. They're systematic and predictable—making us predictably irrational.[18]

And the lessons of behavioral economics apply perfectly to obesity. How else do we explain that after billions spent, we still don't have a program to which people can turn for sustainable weight loss? We don't regain weight because we lack nutrition information. Instead, the weight often returns thanks to early life programming, thinking, habits, and behaviors. Look at it this way. How did your mother comfort you when you were young and didn't feel well or had a tough day at school? I'll bet she gave you something to eat. Millions of us have been conditioned to view food as a reward or treat. And we don't abandon this early life programming in adulthood. Sometimes, it gets worse. A chocolate chip cookie might be a treat for an active ten-year-old gymnast or dancer. But what is that same cookie for a busy, overworked forty-year-old executive with no time to exercise and a history of weight problems?

A recent government report examined behavioral economics' importance in food choices in the context of government food assistance programs, outlining several vital elements in promoting healthy food choices. The authors pointed out that self-control and willpower have little influence on long-term dietary decisions, noting emotion and impulsive behavior's impact instead.[19] I often think that if we could harness these emotions to promote healthier options, it could make a significant contribution to helping reverse the obesity pandemic.

Accepting Reality

So, if behavior plays a major role in food decision-making, how do we overcome that? Rather than looking for a hidden willpower gas tank or deluding ourselves into believing that we can enjoy "all foods in moderation," perhaps we should accept that we are fragile, distractible beings. Our flagging energies and other inconsistencies aren't signs of weakness or a character flaw. They're part of what it means to be human. Think of willpower as an emotion. And like any emotion, it ebbs and flows. No one is happy, sad, or angry all the time. Some days you feel more in control, and others you feel like a bowl of mush. Your will, reasoning powers, and rational decision-making skills will come and go depending on what's happening to you and how you feel.

If willpower and self-control are more akin to emotions than limitless fuel tanks, perhaps we can use them and learn to ride out bad moments. Your feelings aren't a life sentence. I have a patient who joked that if she acted on every feeling or impulse, she'd divorce her husband, abandon her kids, quit her job, and burn down her house. Feelings pass. Tomorrow, joy could easily replace the anger you feel today. Similarly, when you need to perform a challenging task, see your loss of self-control as temporary rather than throwing in the towel and telling yourself you need or deserve a potato chip or Häagen-Dazs break.

The problem here, in weight loss, is that your lack of motivation to succeed can lead to thousands in increased medical costs, damage your health, and a decrease in your quality of life. So, what's the solution? While most people can power through tasks they don't enjoy for a while, weight control is a lifelong endeavor. It never ends. We must find a path to doing things we don't want to do.

Talley's Take: Broadway Blues

If it's true that you are what you eat, then my client Lana, a veteran Broadway performer, is ice cream.

Ever since she was a girl, Lana has loved ice cream. Vanilla, chocolate, butter pecan, chocolate chip mint, cookie dough—name the ice cream, and chances are Lana would eat it. Lana had a bowl of ice cream every afternoon after school for as long as she can remember. Then, on weekends, Lana and her family headed to a local diner for brunch, where she and her siblings had blueberry pancakes and ice cream.

No one saw anything wrong with her ice cream habit. Lana was young and active in dance, gymnastics, and swimming, so, like many kids, she could eat what she wanted and not gain weight.

However, as Lana got older and exercised less, her metabolism slowed and she gained weight. Along the way, Lana never abandoned her childhood ice cream habit.

At age thirty and 60 pounds overweight, she scheduled an emergency appointment with her primary care physician.

"I haven't felt well, doctor," said Lana. "I'm always thirsty. I pee a lot and am always hungry, even after a full meal. I'm also tired, and my vision is blurry. What's wrong with me?" she asked.

"I'm not sure, but given your symptoms and 32 BMI, I think you might be prediabetic, so I'm ordering a full workup," the doctor said.

Prediabetes is when blood glucose or hemoglobin A1C (HbA1C) levels are higher than usual. About 30 percent of prediabetics develop type 2 diabetes within five years. When 33 percent of US adults have prediabetes, this is a condition we shouldn't take lightly.

So, Lana's prediabetes was a concern. But like many chronic illnesses, it's a symptom of something else. Equally concerning to me was Lana's daily ice cream habit—the likely source of her obesity and prediabetes. Depending on the flavor and brand, a pint of ice cream can contain 1,000 calories, more than some people's daily calorie intake in other foods. Keeping up this habit for years can lead to significant weight gain.

Lana turned to ice cream for everything—as a reward or treat after a stressful day at work, as comfort after a fight with a boyfriend, or as a way of feeling less inhibited before an audition or big performance.

Lana's ice cream habit simply confirmed what behavioral psychologists have known for a long time: Stress-related experiences and eating patterns are closely related. When stress is unrelenting, craving rich food such as ice cream can become an almost natural response.

I noticed distinct patterns in Lana's ice cream consumption. She ate ice cream at the same time of day, in the same place, and in the same emotional state. For example, Lana always craved ice cream after waking up around 7 a.m.

I recognized Lana's ice cream obsession for what it was—habituated behavior.

You've likely heard that humans are creatures of habit, unconsciously completing one task after another. Some habits are healthy; others are not. Lana's ice cream obsession fell firmly in the latter category.

As we talked further, I saw a pattern in Lana that all emotional eaters share. Lana wasn't eating because she was hungry. Instead, her hunger was hedonic. The term "hedonic hunger" refers to a preoccupation with and desire to eat for pleasure without physical hunger.

Ice cream helped Lana soothe her uncomfortable emotions. I told her that the desire for ice cream might go away if she tried a blocking behavior. This could be walking, talking on the phone, or simply closing her eyes and breathing deeply for five minutes.

Her reward was comfort. Once you understand the habit, you can change the behavior.

The downside here is that habits are difficult to break, especially pleasure-based habits. Enjoyable behaviors such as eating prompt our brains to release dopamine. If you do something repeatedly, and dopamine is released when you do it, that strengthens the habit even more. And even when you're not doing it, dopamine creates a craving to do it again.

I hate to be the bearer of bad news, but there's no easy formula for changing habits. Likewise, there is no single way of doing so.

We're all different, with unique personalities, experiences, desires, and idiosyncrasies. Best methods for changing patterns vary from person to person.

In Lana's case, blocking behaviors such as talking or texting a friend and walking worked best. But that might not work for you.

What also helped Lana was an ice cream substitute. One of the biggest reasons people fail at weight loss is that they feel deprived after eliminating a food or group of foods. Who wants to feel deprived or like they're missing out? Fortunately, there are great-tasting, low-calorie substitutes for almost every high-fat or high-calorie food. Lana found several ice cream alternatives, including low-calorie frozen fruit and yogurt bars.

Lana and I also talked about ice cream's role in her life. "I don't know how I'm going to survive without ice cream," she told me. I saw my role here as adding some perspective. "Lana, you can have any food you want. However, you may never have the life you want if you keep eating food that causes you to lose control, like ice cream."

I encourage big-picture thinking with clients who have control problems around certain foods. With any food, they need to ask themselves one simple question: "Does this food work for or against me?" Ice cream works against Lana. "True deprivation is eating foods that deprive you of a lifetime of self-control and happiness," I told her.

Most habit changes take time. Sometimes it requires repeated experiments and failures. But once you understand how a habit operates and diagnose the triggers, you can master it.

SECTION
III

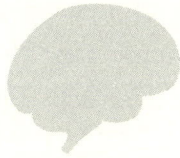

Dr. Lonky's Revolutionary Four-Step Program for Combating the Obesity Epidemic

When I see a new patient, I take a detailed medical history—a record of a person's health. A personal medical history includes information about allergies, surgeries, immunizations, past and current illnesses, a physical exam, and test results. The goal is simple: I need this information to understand the patient's health and determine if anything might direct me toward a proper diagnosis and therapy.

Our approach toward weight management should follow a similar path. What in that person's background caused them to be overweight by 50, 100, or even 200 pounds? I'm almost wasting time telling my heaviest patients to eat less and move more. They know this, but many can't, and a fair percentage don't want to.

Given that obesity diminishes almost every aspect of health, it's easy to turn negative. While putting this book together, I fell into that familiar trap. Still, I knew I couldn't sit still. I needed to do something. We can't control our government or food companies or force billion-dollar corporations to stop polluting our world with endocrine-disrupting chemicals. There is no one-size-fits-all weight-loss book in the works. GLP-1 agonists such as Zepbound™, Ozempic®, and Wegovy®, which have skyrocketed in popularity in the US, show great promise and have helped change the narrative on obesity, but they're an incomplete solution. Mark my words, we will never medicate our way out of the obesity epidemic. No one is coming to save us. We must save ourselves.

While it's obvious the obesity epidemic goes far beyond personal choice, we all have individual agency and, therefore, some control over our behaviors, habits, and decisions related to our overall lifestyle that can contribute to weight gain or obesity.

So, I created a comprehensive yet easy-to-follow program emphasizing individual responsibility, choice, and self-management. I quickly realized such a program could prevent and even reverse the many epigenetic changes that increase our susceptibility to obesity.

AIPE is that program.

AIPE outlines a four-step strategy crafted to guide individuals, regardless of whether they are dealing with obesity, excess weight, or concerns about potential weight gain, through a straightforward and manageable program. Most importantly, I designed it to help those giving birth to the next generation reverse the trends referred to earlier in this book: the persistent weight increases we've seen over the past few decades, including in birth weight. I refer to this four-step plan by the first letters of each step: Accept, Identify, Prevent, and Eliminate—together, AIPE.

A—Accept

The initial letter in the AIPE program is A, and it holds paramount significance among the four. This A signifies Accept, and I want to emphasize that it is the most crucial element. Acknowledging the need for change is the foundational step in any transformation. Acceptance can be challenging; I understand that. Many individuals grappling with excess weight often fail to recognize they have a problem or are hesitant to admit it. According to a recent Gallup poll, more than half of US adults (55 percent) don't think they are overweight and aren't trying to shed pounds.

For obesity, acceptance means coming to grips with two things: toxic compounds and toxic behaviors.

TOXIC COMPOUNDS

From the moment of conception, we are enveloped by tens of thousands of toxic compounds. These substances, often from various sources such as the environment, food, and everyday products, create a pervasive backdrop that influences our overall well-being. We must accept that we are victims of toxic compound exposures. Acceptance doesn't mean you'll immediately rid yourself of toxic chemicals, those endocrine disrupters that cause epigenetic changes. However, you can't do anything until you accept that you carry this body burden.

TOXIC BEHAVIORS

Second, as adults, we often find ourselves entangled in a web of unhealthy behaviors that significantly contribute to the challenges we face in maintaining a healthy weight. Do you eat when you're bored or stressed? Do you eat when you're angry or upset? Do you negotiate with foods you always overeat? Do you shop for groceries when you're hungry? Other behaviors, cultivated over time, may also include poor dietary choices, sedentary lifestyles, irregular sleep patterns, and coping mechanisms such as emotional eating. A combination of societal norms, stress, and modern life's demands frequently influences the adoption of these habits.

If any of this sounds familiar to you, you must accept that the problem isn't food. It's your toxic thinking and behavior around food. Rolls, cookies, and candy bars don't have any real control over you. They only have the power we give them. Patients frequently ask me about the best diet for weight loss. My answer is always the same: Your diet is secondary. It matters, and it doesn't. The most important factor for taking charge of your relationship with food is accepting that toxic thinking and behaviors are holding you back.

ACCEPTANCE IS THE FIRST STEP TO BETTER

You must accept that you're carrying a burden of toxic compounds and behaviors because doing so is the only way to get better. As the author Bryant McGill observed, "Acceptance is the road to all change." However, it's important not to confuse acceptance with resignation, even though they are often grouped together. Resignation is accompanied by thoughts such as "I simply have to endure the situation and make the best of it." This mindset can make you feel trapped, victim to a circumstance or situation, and powerless to effect change. Unfortunately, there's a common misconception that acceptance means surrendering to a situation, regardless of how challenging it may be. Even the reputable Oxford Dictionary seems to misinterpret acceptance, defining it as "Willingness to tolerate a difficult situation: a mood of resigned acceptance."

Acceptance involves recognizing that a situation is what it is and acknowledging that there's a path forward. While you may be contending with a load of toxic compounds, thoughts, and behaviors, it doesn't imply that you are destined for a lifetime of weight problems and poor health. Embracing the fact that there is a problem is not surrender; I might even propose the term "acknowledgment" for a clearer understanding. Accepting that you've gained 100 pounds in five years and understanding that there are steps you can take to address it marks the starting point of liberation and the journey toward positive change.

I once heard acceptance described as "recognizing the truth of this moment without resistance." That's an apt definition. The truth could be that you're obese, harboring toxic chemicals, and engaging in unhealthy behaviors and habits that worsen your weight problems. There's nothing wrong with admitting any of this. It doesn't mean you're crazy, dumb, or damaged in some way. It simply means that you're in a predicament facing over 200 million US citizens. You're in good company.

Acceptance is not something you can grasp solely by reading a book, watching a video, or listening to a self-help guru. It is a profoundly personal and experiential facet of life that extends beyond mere theoretical comprehension. Think of a time when you felt profoundly accepting—releasing the need for control and accepting life's ups and downs, or surrendering to what you can't change and focusing on those things within your control.

While acceptance—much like resignation—involves recognizing a lack of power or control, it doesn't stop there. Unlike the passive experience of resignation, acceptance is an active state, one in which you can commit to making things better by:

1. Acknowledging the reality of your situation (That's the only way to transform it.)

2. Embracing your thoughts and feelings (Don't fight them.)

3. Identifying your sense of agency (You're not powerless.)

4. Seeking support and guidance (Use AIPE.)

This acceptance approach, as I like to call it, offers the possibility of preventing obesity by limiting or avoiding pollutants and exposure, especially in pregnant women and babies. Acceptance applies equally to your behavior around food, especially the foods that are at the root of your weight problems.

I frequently remind my patients that we all have these terrible relationships with food and eating. However, those who fight that reality lessen their chances of lasting success if weight loss is the goal. But if you are willing to accept that you harbor these behaviors, it's not a time to feel guilty. Instead, it's a time to rejoice. You've taken the first and most crucial step in managing and perhaps even preventing obesity. No wonder A is the first letter of the alphabet.

I—Identify

The next step is identifying and locating the toxic compounds in your life that are potential causes of weight gain. The challenge here, of course, is that there are almost too many to count. According to the consumer resource Environmental Working Group, about fifty chemicals or chemical classes have earned the obesogen designation. But fifty is undoubtedly a conservative estimate. Just living our everyday lives exposes us to dozens of toxic compounds.

If you smoke, drink alcohol, or lead a generally unhealthy lifestyle, it's a safe bet that you have high exposure to environmental toxins. On the other hand, even the healthiest people come into regular contact with obesogens.

Here are just a few examples of obesogen-containing products we consume or use:

- Low-fat and sugar-free foods

- Commercially raised meat and dairy products

- Highly processed and preserved foods

- Plastic water bottles and storage containers

- Pesticides

- Plastic toys

- Makeup and skincare products

- Shampoos and hair care products

- Soaps, detergents, and other laundry products

- Dry cleaning agents

- Household cleaners

- Deodorants

- Flame retardants (applied to furniture and children's clothes)

I know this is a big list. Chemicals are added to these products because they serve a purpose. Regardless, they could be contributing to your weight problem.

After accepting the reality of our body's chemical burden, we must identify the toxins we're exposed to so we can do something about it. But first, we need to know what to look for.

Here are six types of obesogens that concern me:

1. **Bisphenols** are a group of chemical compounds widely used in producing plastics and other materials. One of the most well-known and widely used bisphenols is bisphenol A (BPA). Bisphenols are commonly used to manufacture polycarbonate plastics, epoxy resins, and other products due to their strength and durability.

2. **Phthalates** are chemical compounds commonly used as plasticizers, which are added to plastics to increase their flexibility, durability, and transparency. They are also used in other products, including personal care items, cosmetics, medical devices, and more. Phthalates are not chemically bound to the plastics or products they're added to, which means they can leach out over time and potentially be released into the environment or absorbed by the body.

3. **Atrazine** is an herbicide primarily used to control broadleaf and grassy weeds in crops such as corn, sugarcane, and sorghum. Atrazine is known for its effectiveness in preventing weed growth by inhibiting photosynthesis in plants.

4. **Organotins** are a class of chemical compounds that contain tin atoms bonded to organic (carbon-containing) groups. These compounds have been used for various industrial and commercial purposes due to their unique stability, durability, and antifungal properties.

5. **Perfluorooctanoic acid** (PFOA), or C8, is a synthetic chemical used in various industrial and commercial applications. It belongs to a class of per- and polyfluoroalkyl substances (PFAS), known for their strong chemical bonds and heat, water, and oil resistance. PFOA is part of a larger group of PFAS compounds that have similar properties. They are used in non-stick cookware.

6. **Parabens** are a class of synthetic chemicals commonly used as preservatives in a wide range of personal care, cosmetic, and pharmaceutical products to extend their shelf life by preventing the growth of microbes such as bacteria, yeast, and mold. They are valued for their antimicrobial properties and ability to maintain product integrity.

1. BISPHENOL-A (BPA)

BPA is a synthetic compound that makes polycarbonate plastics and resins that line food and beverage cans. Other BPA-containing products include:

- Toiletries

- Menstrual products

- Thermal printer receipts

- Household electronics

- Eyeglass lenses

- Sports equipment

- Dental filling sealants

BPA is similar in structure to estradiol, the primary female sex hormone. This structural similarity allows BPA to bind to estrogen receptors in the body, potentially affecting various physiological processes. This binding process may induce insulin resistance, inflammation, oxidative stress, and fat cell formation. Humans are exposed to BPA when eating food stored or reheated in BPA-lined containers. Because the compound isn't fully attached to plastic, it can easily leach into your food. BPA doesn't discriminate—it exists in newborns, children, and adults. In addition, we can measure it in bodily fluids and tissues such as blood, urine, saliva, breast milk, and fatty tissue.

What You Can Do about BPA

- Buy reusable water bottles; avoid plastic water bottles.

- Limit your use of canned and packaged foods (if you can't limit canned foods, rinse them thoroughly).

- Microwave your food in glass containers.

- Choose electronic receipts, boarding passes, or movie tickets when possible. If you get paper receipts, try to avoid putting them in your pocket.

- Store leftovers in glass or stainless steel containers instead of plastic.

---

2. PHTHALATES

Phthalates are a group of manufactured chemicals used to make plastics more durable and flexible. We find them in toys, medical devices, food packaging, detergents, soaps, shampoo, nail polish, lotions, and perfumes. Di(2-ethylhexyl) phthalate (DEHP) is the most common phthalate. It binds to androgen receptors, impairing testosterone attachment to cells and producing anti-androgenic effects that may contribute to obesity. In addition, as some research has shown, phthalates may affect peroxisome proliferator–activated receptors (PPARs), a group of nuclear receptor proteins that play a crucial role in regulating various metabolic processes, including lipid and glucose metabolism. This interaction could contribute to metabolic changes and have implications for obesity.

Phthalates have been investigated for their effects on cell signaling pathways involved in metabolism, such as those related to adipogenesis (the process of forming fat cells) and glucose homeostasis (maintaining stable blood sugar levels). Obesity and related metabolic disorders are closely linked to these pathways.

Food and drink are the primary forms of phthalate exposure. Dust is also a significant exposure source.

Studies in children have linked these compounds to increased body mass index (BMI) and obesity. Phthalates are ubiquitous, and their metabolites—or end products—have been detected in over 75 percent of the US population.

What You Can Do about Phthalates

- Avoid fast food when possible.

- Stay clear of PVC-made plastic wrap and plastic food containers that carry the recycling label Number 3. Choose glass or stainless steel food containers instead.

- Reheat food or beverages in glass containers. Many plastic containers contain phthalates, and heating increases their release into the food.

- Read labels and avoid cosmetics and personal care products that contain phthalates.

3. ATRAZINE

Atrazine is a widely used herbicide found in US streams, rivers, and lakes near fields, especially in spring and summer. Though drinking water is not a frequent source of human exposure, atrazine is one of the most commonly found pesticides in surface and ground waters. The small amounts in waterways become incorporated into algae and are then eaten by fish, which we then consume. Because it's applied to crops used as livestock feed, milk and meat also contain atrazine residues.

Like BPA and phthalates, atrazine has anti-androgenic and -estrogenic effects. It also reduces the production of luteinizing hormone, a hormone involved in sexual development and functioning. In addition, animal studies show that long-term atrazine exposure may increase obesity and insulin resistance risk, especially when linked to high-fat diets. Although there's a suggestion that atrazine might lead to weight gain, research hasn't definitively confirmed this. Translating findings from animal studies to human health is complex and seldom straightforward.

What You Can Do about Atrazine

- An affordable, high-quality activated carbon/carbon block filter removes atrazine and other herbicides from drinking water. You can even buy pitchers with built-in carbon filters that will do this.

- Avoid digging or working in soils where herbicide containing atrazine has been applied.

- Ensure that those applying atrazine are trained in proper application techniques to minimize drift and runoff. This includes using appropriate equipment, calibrating sprayers, and avoiding application during windy or rainy conditions.

- Support farming practices prioritizing soil health, biodiversity, and reduced chemical inputs. Sustainable agriculture methods can help create healthier ecosystems and reduce the need for intensive herbicide use.

4. ORGANOTINS

Organotins are a class of industrial compounds used as polyvinyl chloride (PVC) stabilizers, antifouling paints, and pesticides. One of them is called tributyltin (TBT), an active ingredient in antifungal paint applied to boats and ships to prevent the growth of marine organisms on the hull. Unfortunately, it's released into the water and deposited in sediments, contaminating many lakes and coastal waters. Again, smaller water species entrap this chemical, and it works its way up the food chain.

In 2018, researchers discovered that marine waters contaminated with TBT could stimulate fat cell formation while reducing muscle mass.[1] Human exposure most likely occurs through dietary sources like contaminated seafood and shellfish, or for the people handling these products, through the skin.

What You Can Do about Organotins

- As exposure to organotins is primarily through shellfish and fish consumption, it is worth checking with your healthcare professional about the amount and frequency of your seafood consumption and the types of fish and shellfish you should consume. Since organotins have been detected in seafood due to their persistence in the environment, consider sustainably sourced seafood, which can indirectly contribute to reducing the demand for antifouling paints that release organotins into the oceans.

- If you own a boat or marine equipment, avoid using antifouling paints that contain organotins.

- Read labels and avoid polyvinyl chloride (PVC or vinyl) plastic products. Select household items, clothing, and consumer goods labeled "organotin-free" or "TBT-free."

- Minimize your use of other plastic and foam products when possible.

5. PERFLUOROOCTANOIC ACID (PFOA) AND PERFLUOROOCTANE SULFONIC ACID (PFOS)

PFOA and PFOS are part of the per- and polyfluoroalkyl substances (PFAS) chemical group. They are both difficult to break down in the environment and the human body. Contaminated water is one of the sources of human PFOA exposure. In addition, PFOA helps make furniture and carpeting spill-resistant, so babies that crawl around on these surfaces and then put their hands in their mouths have yet another source. And, of course, non-stick cookware is a source.

Once ingested, it can remain in your body for long periods. Like phthalates, PFOA activates PPAR receptors in your body, which are involved in fat metabolism. Based on experimental data, scientists have concluded that prenatal PFOA exposure increases children's risk of adult-onset obesity.[2]

What to Do about PFOA and PFOS

- Be aware of food packaging that contains grease-repellent coatings. Examples include microwave popcorn bags and fast-food wrappers and boxes.

- It's best to avoid stain resistant carpets or furniture. You might hate me now after your kids spill grape juice on your new couch, but you'll thank me later.

- Avoid clothing, luggage, camping, and sports equipment treated for water or stain resistance.

- Reduce or avoid the use of non-stick cookware. Stop using products if non-stick coatings show signs of wear.

---

6. PARABENS

Many products, such as cosmetics, moisturizers, hair-care products, and shaving creams, contain parabens. The skin absorbs parabens from these products. Parabens also can enter the body when we swallow or eat paraben-containing pharmaceuticals, foods, and drinks.

The use of butylparaben-containing cosmetics during pregnancy may increase childhood obesity risk. A potential link has been observed between increased levels of butylparaben in mothers' urine and higher BMI in their children, especially among daughters, until their eighth birthday.[3] Also, parabens may cause epigenetic changes that damage satiety signaling and interfere with appetite regulation.

What to Do about Parabens

- Reduce your exposure to parabens by reading the ingredient label on the back of food product packaging. Look for words ending in "paraben" such as methylparaben, propylparaben, ethylparaben, and so on. Many food products, including beer, sauces, desserts, soft drinks, jams, pickles, frozen dairy products, processed vegetables, and flavoring syrups, use parabens for preservation.

- Many products that contain fragrance also contain parabens. Fragrance can be a catch-all term for various undisclosed chemicals. Opt for fragrance-free products or those scented with natural essential oils. Also, look for personal care products labeled "paraben-free" and read ingredient lists on labels to avoid parabens.

- Consider using natural and organic products, as they are less likely to contain synthetic preservatives like parabens. Look for products certified by reputable organic or natural certification organizations.

- Consider limiting your use of products that stay on your skin for extended periods, like lotions and creams, as they can lead to greater paraben absorption.

- Babies and young children are particularly sensitive to chemical exposure. Choose paraben-free products for them as well.

IDENTIFYING TOXIC EATING BEHAVIORS

I have a patient who eats whenever she feels overwhelmed. If she has too many work projects, is exhausted from caring for her elderly mother, or argues with her teenage daughters, she turns to food. I have another patient who binges on Oreo cookies whenever an uncomfortable emotion surfaces, and one who'll eat an entire pizza when bored.

My patients know that emotional eating is their Achilles' heel. They know what they're doing and see it's not serving them. Yet, they keep doing it and can't seem to break the cycle. Here's why. *Synaptic plasticity*, a process central to learning, memory, and the development of repetitive behaviors such as habits, involves modifying the strength of connections (synapses) between neurons in the brain. When we repeat a behavior over time, the neural pathways associated with that behavior become more efficient, making it easier for the behavior to be triggered and executed in the future. I think of it as "neurons that fire together, wire together."

It's easy to see why my patients can't stop their destructive eating behaviors—they're neurologically ingrained. The thought of leaving behind these old habits and creating new ones frightens and overwhelms them. As one patient said, "If I can't turn to my oatmeal cookie, what will I do to comfort myself when I'm upset?" The good news for my patients is that they're not in denial about these toxic eating behaviors. They have taken the first step. In the next step, it's important to recognize and pinpoint unhealthy eating behaviors. I advise my patients to list these behaviors that hinder their well-being. Maintaining this list in a journal or incorporating it into a vision board proves beneficial for them as a constructive step toward implementing enduring changes and embracing healthier eating habits.

Of course, healthy eating is a relative term. No food is "healthy" if you overeat it. Also, healthy eating extends well beyond food choice.

Every person I know understands that an ideal diet consists of fruits, vegetables, low-fat dairy, and lean protein. However, healthy eating habits also include how you eat: how you fill your plate, how you eat your food, and when you eat. Healthy eating habits equal healthy eating. It's that simple. Look at your eating habits and see if you can identify which ones serve your health and which do not. Understanding that some of your habits encourage unhealthy eating is an excellent first step.

Do you feel guilty about eating?

"I can't believe I ate that. I feel so guilty."

Guilt is one of the most common emotions in people with weight issues. I don't know of anyone who hasn't experienced it. A 2019 survey found that one-third of all food Americans eat makes them feel guilty. An awareness of unhealthy food causes most food guilt.[4] High sugar content and overeating are also leading causes of shame. Internally, feeling guilt is often seen as something productive. We beat ourselves up and tell ourselves to do better for our own sake. However, the guilt we feel only does harm.

Guilt arises when a person feels they've done something wrong. Sneaking a Twinkie or Hershey's bar isn't the same as stealing, hurting someone, being rude, lying, or cheating. It's appropriate to feel guilty if you hurt someone or lie. However, you're not born knowing there's anything wrong with lying or stealing. You're taught right from wrong.

Unfortunately, these same beliefs are taught regarding food. We hear again and again about good and bad foods. The experts tell us a particular food is unhealthy and will make us sick, so we shouldn't eat it. Just as we're taught morals and values, we're taught guilt, including food guilt. It's a learned behavior.

I have some news for you. Food is indifferent—it's not moral or immoral. It can't betray or deceive you. It only has the power you give it. There are no good or bad foods. There are only good or bad relationships with food. A "bad" food is a food that causes you to lose control and overeat. But that food might not be a problem for your friend or spouse. I overeat ice cream. My wife doesn't. Ice cream isn't bad for her, but it's not a good choice for me.

The idea here is that all foods are morally equivalent. Don't view them as good or bad. Instead, ask yourself, "Does this food work for me and my control?" That's the only way to evaluate food. What's worse—breaking the diet or beating yourself up about it? We eat to live. It shouldn't come with so much guilt.

Do you obsess over calories?

Calories count, but what's more important than the calories in a cookie or roll is how many cookies or rolls you eat. If you can limit yourself to a single 50-calorie roll before dinner, then you're OK. However, if that single, 50-calorie roll stirs cravings, it could quickly turn into thousands of calories. So, think about how much you eat of a particular food rather than the calories in that food.

Do you ignore your body's hunger cues?

Hunger is complex, and your body produces more than a dozen hormones that promote or suppress it. Tips for tricking, outsmarting, or hacking our hunger hormones abound, but this implies we have control over these hormones. Your stomach and adipose tissue produce the best-known hunger hormones, ghrelin and leptin. These hormones regulate your body's appetite, tell your brain when you're hungry, and signal your brain when you're full.

Because ghrelin is a "short-acting" hormone, what you ate yesterday doesn't affect it. And if you ignore hunger, ghrelin levels will continue to rise, triggering out-of-control eating. Many people believe—often as a side effect of dieting—that they should fear or suppress hunger. However, hunger, like thirst, is a natural biological cue that helps keep us alive. Early signs of hunger often include an empty feeling in the stomach or growling sounds. But suppose you ignore your body's early hunger cues. In that case, perhaps because you're busy or simply don't trust that you need to eat—or if those cues have gone silent from years of denying them, you may become dizzy, lightheaded, headachy, irritable, or unable to focus or concentrate. Ideally, you should notice and respond to earlier signs of hunger before you reach this point.

Do you yo-yo diet?

Let's put all our cards on the table: Yo-yo dieting is terrible for your weight and health. A study that followed more than 150,000 women for eleven years found that for adult women, yo-yo dieting or weight cycling can increase their risk for coronary heart disease and cardiac arrest.[5] In addition, weight cycling can increase body fat percentage and stimulate muscle loss. Also, weight gain cycles increase fatty liver disease risk. Yo-yo dieting can also lead to disordered eating habits and long-term weight struggles. Finally, for people with diabetes, yo-yo dieting can disrupt blood glucose management.

Bottom line: There's nothing good about yo-yo dieting. Don't do it.

Do you go into food situations hungry?

Do you grocery shop on an empty stomach? Do you starve yourself all day before a celebratory meal or before going out to dinner? Going into food situations hungry is like throwing a match to gasoline. You're starving, and your neuropeptide-Y levels are dropping while your ghrelin levels are rising, so you're far more likely to fall off the wagon.

Do you gravitate to the latest diet fad?

Research has shown that dieters typically lose 5 to 10 percent of their starting weight in the first six months. After that, however, at least one-third to two-thirds of dieters regain more weight than they lost within four or five years, no matter what program they follow.[6] They fail, say psychologist Kima Cargill and anthropologist Janet Chrzan in their book, *Anxious Eaters*, because these diets are not really about food. "They're about identity, status, control, and transformation. They have power because we believe they will fulfill our desires for self-improvement," say the authors.[7]

Do you keep going back to foods you overeat?

If you have a history of overeating French fries, don't delude yourself into believing that this is a food you can bargain with and come out on top. You'll get fleeced—and fat—every time.

Do you eat late at night?

Late-night eating impairs sleep, increases hunger, reduces calorie burn, and can change the metabolism of obese adults. In addition, late-night eating also increases fat storage.

Do you eat too fast?

It can take twenty minutes for your brain to realize that your body has had enough to eat. Scarfing down a burger at your desk while you work or text may cause the meal to go by so quickly that your stomach cannot send satiety signals to your brain. Eating food too fast can have you eating more than you should.

Do you overload your plate?

Research shows that people eat more from fuller plates, even without hunger. People are finishers. Most are loathe to leave food on their plate, especially if they're dining out at a nice restaurant. Dialing in the right portion size is an excellent way to improve your eating habits. It's better to put too little rather than too much on your plate. You can always come back for seconds.

Do you skip meals?

Skipping meals is an unhealthy eating habit. It can lead to binge eating, over-indulging, and excessive snacking. Plus, you can end up so hungry that you make bad choices. So, instead, establish a regular eating schedule.

Do you only eat one type of food at meals?

No one wants to be bored at meals. However, studies show that food variety—multiple foods or sensory characteristics within and across meals—stimulates consumption.[8] Still, enjoying a wide range of foods and eating a healthy diet is possible. Fruits, vegetables, whole grains, and a moderate amount of unsaturated fats, meat, and dairy can help you maintain a steady weight. In addition, various healthy, nutritious foods leave less room for high-sugar, high-fat foods. The key here is never to go hungry.

Do you eat when you aren't hungry?

This one is pretty straightforward. If you aren't hungry, you shouldn't eat. But we often eat out of boredom because there's something tasty in the break room or even because we saw a tempting TV commercial for a favorite food. Snacking for the sake of snacking is a bad eating habit.

GETTING STARTED

You don't have to be a chemist or toxicologist or hold a PhD in nutrition to identify the chemicals, behaviors, and habits contributing to your weight problems. But you do need to be honest, especially with yourself.

Start with your day-to-day life. For example, do you regularly use products loaded with endocrine-disrupting chemicals? Do you use skincare products containing parabens? Do you store food in glass or plastic? Do you remove your dry cleaning from the plastic bag before hanging it in the closet? Together, these practices could contribute to your weight problems. And remember, when it comes to environmental compounds in our homes, it's not just us but also our children who are impacted by these toxic exposures.

Becoming aware of the thought patterns, eating habits, and behaviors at the root of most weight problems is equally critical. You can begin by thinking about the role of food in your life. Are you programmed to view food as a "treat" or "goodie"? Do you reward yourself with cookies or potato chips after a hard day? Do you eat out of boredom or stress? Have you been deluding yourself into believing that achieving and maintaining a healthy weight involves discipline or willpower? Do you negotiate with foods you have a history of overeating? Changing your thinking, habits, and behaviors is far more critical, especially in the presence of foods you have a long history of overeating. That's the importance of the Identify component of AIPE.

P—Prevent

Why do doctors talk about prevention? Because preventing an illness is nearly always easier than treating it. Prevention is so powerful that a cardiologist colleague once told me he'd lose 90 percent of his business if his patients simply adopted healthier lifestyle habits. "It's much better to recommend heart-healthy foods, exercise, and stress management than to perform a cardiac catheterization," he said. But sadly, his business is thriving. Part of the problem lies in medicine. Modern medicine focuses on injury or illness treatment, not prevention.

Once you've **Accepted** the current situation and **Identified** the toxic chemicals and behaviors holding you back, your next goal is to **Prevent** them from wreaking havoc on your health. To that end, I have both good and bad news. I'll give you the bad news first. If you're an obese adult, then prevention can feel like closing the barn door after the horses have escaped. You carry a body burden of synthetic chemicals and pollutants, and they've been there for a long time. The good news is that preventing further absorption of these chemicals will give your body time to remove them (you'll need some help and time, which I explain in the next section, Eliminate). Preventing absorption while reducing exposure is critical because these chemicals harm us and affect our children's future health and development, and even that of our grandchildren and great-grandchildren. Toxic chemicals' impact on generations long after direct exposure to these contaminants occurred is real. Therefore, prevention should have a particular resonance for pregnant women or women and couples planning to conceive.

BABY STEPS: WHERE TO BEGIN

The food we eat, the water we drink, the air we breathe, and many household items we use daily contain environmental toxins. They're invisible, and most exposures go undetected. Also, it's not the occasional exposure that concerns me. It's the cumulative effect of repeated exposures over many years. In addition, the growth in industrial manufacturing, fossil fuel consumption, and chemical-intensive crop production have dramatically changed the scale and complexity of humans' environmental toxin exposures. Unfortunately, you won't avoid toxic exposures altogether—it's impossible.

But that doesn't mean you're powerless. Strategies to prevent your body's absorption of toxicants found in your food, home, or workspace can be as simple as adding "binders" such as activated charcoal and certain herbs like cilantro to your diet.

Be careful with cleaning products

It's hard to believe, but some commonly used household cleaners could make us overweight, especially children, by altering our gut microbiota (the bacteria in our gut). These products release dangerous chemicals, including volatile organic compounds (VOCs). Even natural fragrances such as citrus and lavender can react to produce hazardous indoor pollutants. Rather than tell you what to buy, I have some general guidelines for what to avoid, if possible. Here's my list:

- Formaldehyde

- Ammonia

- Triclosan

- Sodium laureth sulfate

- Phthalates

- Propylene glycol

- 2-Butoxyethanol

- Parabens

- Sodium hydroxide

- Chlorine

- Phosphates

- Sulfate1,4-Dioxane

- Ammonium

- Tetrachloroethylene

- Methylisothiazolinone

- Ethanolamine

- Triethanolamine

- Diethanolamine

- Quaternium-15

- Triclocarban

a. **Ammonia** is toxic when inhaled, swallowed, or touched. Never mix bleach or any bleach-containing product with any cleaner containing ammonia. The gases created from this combination can lead to chronic breathing problems and even death.

b. Many **antibacterial products and disinfectants** contain ingredients ranging from bleach to hormone-disrupting triclosan. The truth is that these products are rarely needed. Honestly, soap and water will usually do the trick. There are natural options, too. Just read the label before you buy.

c. **Glycol ethers** are common in most general cleaners and may harm your nervous system, liver, and kidneys.

d. **Chlorine bleach** is strong, corrosive, and irritating to the eyes, skin, and lungs. Bleach also stains clothes. Why bother with it?

e. Many cleaning products contain **petroleum solvents** (watch for this term on ingredient lists). Again, read labels before you buy and look for cleaning products without these ingredients.

f. You might have heard that excessive **phosphate** levels in aquatic environments can harm marine life. Phosphates are essential nutrients for plant growth, including algae. While some level of phosphates is necessary for a healthy aquatic ecosystem, excess phosphates (often from human activities like agricultural runoff, sewage discharge, and the use of phosphate-containing detergents) can lead to *eutrophication*, which occurs when there is an overabundance of nutrients, particularly nitrogen, and phosphorus, in a water body. Although dietary phosphate is essential for bone and tooth development, excessive intake can adversely affect human health. It can lead to conditions such as diarrhea and organ and soft tissue calcification (hardening) while disrupting the body's use of vital minerals like iron, calcium, magnesium, and zinc. Notably, many laundry and dish detergents include phosphate as an ingredient.

g. Hormone-disruptive **phthalates** are common in synthetic fragrances. That lavender bathroom spray might smell great, but it's not good for you. Avoid scented candles and cleaners. Choose phthalate-free products.

h. Other common endocrine-disrupting cleaning product ingredients I suggest you avoid whenever possible are—

- **Cyclosiloxanes** (e.g., hexamethylcyclotrisiloxane, dodecamethylcyclohexylsiloxane)

- **Alkylphenols** (e.g., nonylphenols, octylphenols)

- **Ethanolamides** (e.g., monoethanolamine, diethanolamine)

Eight Alternatives to Toxic Cleaning Products

Cleaning products free from harmful chemicals can contribute to a healthier living environment. Below are eight alternatives and strategies for utilizing cleaning products that are gentler on your body and the environment.

1. **Homemade Cleaning Solutions**

   • Use basic household ingredients like vinegar, baking soda, lemon juice, and castile soap to create many effective cleaning solutions. These ingredients are non-toxic and eco-friendly.

   • Mix equal parts water and white vinegar in a spray bottle for an all-purpose cleaner. You can also add a few drops of essential oil for a pleasant scent.

   • Baking soda makes for a gentle abrasive cleaner and deodorizer. Combine it with water to form a paste for scrubbing.

2. **Plant-Based and Biodegradable Cleaners**

   • Look for cleaning products that are labeled as "plant-based," "biodegradable," or "eco-friendly." These products often use ingredients derived from natural sources that are safer for the environment.

   • Check the ingredient list to ensure no harsh chemicals or synthetic fragrances exist.

3. **Products with Third-Party Certifications**

   • Some cleaning products carry third-party certifications that indicate their safety and environmental friendliness. Look for labels like "EcoLogo," "Green Seal," or "USDA Certified Biobased."

continued

4. **Microfiber Cloths and Reusable Cleaning Tools**

- Microfiber cloths are highly effective at cleaning surfaces with just water, reducing the need for chemical cleaners.

- Use washable and reusable cleaning tools like mops, dusters, and cleaning cloths to minimize waste.

5. **Steam Cleaning**

- Steam cleaning uses heat and moisture to clean and sanitize surfaces. It's an effective method for removing dirt and grime without chemicals.

6. **Hydrogen Peroxide**

- Hydrogen peroxide is a natural disinfectant and can be used to clean and sanitize surfaces. It's a safer alternative to bleach.

7. **Essential Oils**

- Some essential oils, like tea tree and lavender oil, have natural antibacterial properties. Adding drops to your cleaning solutions can provide a pleasant scent and enhance cleaning effectiveness.

8. **Reduce, Reuse, and Recycle**

- Minimize the need for heavy cleaning by maintaining a tidy living environment. Regular tidying reduces the accumulation of dirt and grime.

- Opt for reusable cleaning tools and containers to reduce waste.

Remember that while using non-toxic cleaning products is beneficial, following proper cleaning practices is also important to maintain a healthy and hygienic living space. Always ensure adequate ventilation when cleaning, regardless of the products you use.

And cleaning products aren't the only chemical materials you should watch out for. Regrettably, synthetic chemicals in everyday products such as plastics and fragrances also pose a threat, as these substances can imitate hormones and disrupt our finely tuned endocrine system—the network of hormones and glands that govern our bodies. While commonly associated with puberty, the endocrine system significantly influences all stages of development, metabolism, and behavior. Exposure to synthetic chemicals is a daily occurrence, with heightened vulnerability during crucial developmental phases, such as pregnancy and childhood. However, there are steps we can take to minimize risk. Here are a few ways to protect yourself.

1. Grab a mop. Lead, pesticides, and flame-retardant particles are present in dust. Sweeping or dusting may spread toxins into the air instead of removing them from your home. If you use a vacuum, use one with a HEPA filter.

2. Don't spray bugs and weeds. If you're a gardener, you know how frustrating it can be to rid your plants of pests and weeds. However, avoid pesticides and toxic chemicals that kill these unwanted visitors whenever possible. Pesticides commonly found in bug repellents can affect female hormone production, possibly negatively impacting reproductive health. Problematic ingredients used in bug spray and repellents include DEET, cyfluthrin, permethrin, and pyrethroid. Bug sprays and repellents may also contain hormone-disrupting

chemicals such as parabens, sulfates, phthalates, and synthetic fragrances. To limit exposure, use safe and non-toxic products when possible. Look for products with a "MADE SAFE" label. Avoid using chemical tick-and-flea collars or dips for your pets.

3. Avoid dry-cleaning clothes. Most cleaners use a chemical called perchloroethylene (PERC), which can pollute the air in your home. Use water instead, including on clothes labeled "dry clean only." Hand wash them or ask your dry cleaner to wet clean them. If you must dry clean your clothes, remove them from the plastic bags before bringing them into your home. The plastic is apparently to protect the item while it is in transit. However, the chemicals used in dry cleaning, including dioxin, must be ventilated rather than trapped in the bag.

4. Be careful with oil-based paints, especially spray paints. In 1978, the federal government banned the commercial use of oil-based paint. However, oil-based paints still contain some heavy metals in the pigments. In addition, oil-based paint fumes contain potentially toxic hydrocarbons and high levels of volatile organic compounds (VOCs), which perform numerous functions in paint and evaporate as it dries. The most significant health effects of oil-based paint are from polluted air from VOCs.

5. Look out for flame retardants. Many everyday household items such as couches, carpet padding, and electronics use synthetic flame retardants known to cause metabolic and liver problems that can lead to insulin resistance, which is a significant cause of obesity. To avoid flame retardants, check

furniture labels. Only choose furniture labeled "contains no added flame retardants." Avoiding kids' products made with polyurethane foam is also a good idea. Finally, wash your hands regularly to reduce exposure to products in your home. Cleanliness counts! Wash hands, especially those of young children, often to keep dust from attaching to food or fingers and being consumed.

6. Be careful with cosmetics. It's hard to believe that makeup might make us fat. However, a recent study of 231 cosmetics found perfluoroalkyl and polyfluoroalkyl substances (PFAS) present in more than half, including foundations, mascara, and lip products.[9] PFAS, like other endocrine-disrupting compounds, are lipophilic, so the body stores them in fat tissue. They can persist in the body and exert cumulative effects. When choosing nail polish, avoid products containing dibutyl phthalate, toluene, formaldehyde resin, and camphor. Avoid paraben-containing cosmetics and body care products if you're pregnant or planning on getting pregnant. A study published in *Nature Communications* found that children are likely to become overweight or obese if their mothers are exposed to high paraben levels while pregnant.[10]

BINDERS

Now you have some strategies for avoiding toxic compounds and behaviors. However, changing your behavior, cleaning up your diet, and keeping toxic products out of your home isn't enough, especially if you're already obese. Yes, the human body has an incredible built-in detox system. However, accumulating harmful compounds and acute or repeated toxic exposures can overwhelm even the healthiest person. So, your body might need some help. I recommend gut binders, which bind and remove toxins via the digestive tract, preventing the body from absorbing them.

Binders can help remove the following:

- Heavy metals, including aluminum, mercury, and lead

- Mycotoxins from mold

- Plastic particles containing a myriad of chemical toxins

- Pesticides and herbicides

- Volatile organic compounds (VOCs)

- BPA

- Perfluorinated Compounds (PFAS)

How Binders Work

Binders attach to the toxins to facilitate elimination without recirculation risk. Binders can also help prevent inflammatory reactions and reduce detox symptoms. Take binders at night with lots of water. You may consider adding liver support products such as milk thistle or glutathione if you take activated charcoal.

I have just one caveat. Never start any detox program or take any product without first speaking with a qualified medical professional. I live by the expression, *If it's powerful enough to heal, it's powerful enough to harm.*

So, which binders help prevent the absorption of which chemicals? Here's my list.

Chlorella

Chlorella is a blue-green algae rich in vitamins, minerals, amino acids, and omega-3 fatty acids.

It binds to heavy metals, pesticides, herbicides, mycotoxins, and VOCs. Many detox agents also bind to and remove beneficial minerals and nutrients. However, chlorella only binds to toxins and won't excrete essential minerals and nutrients, so you can use it long-term. It's safe and well-tolerated for most people and can even serve as a multivitamin because of its rich nutrient content. I like it because you can start slowly and build up.

Activated Charcoal

Activated charcoal is a finely ground black powder made from carbon-based organic matter—usually coconut shells, bamboo, or peat. The ingredients are heated at high temperatures and combined with oxygen to "activate" the charcoal, significantly increasing its ability to soak up and remove toxins as it passes through the digestive tract. Charcoal is a "broad-spectrum binder" that eliminates both toxins and helpful minerals and nutrients. I don't recommend long-term activated charcoal use because it can cause mineral depletion. Take it for a few days, and then take a few weeks off.

Clays

There are many clay types on the market, but zeolite and bentonite clays are the gold standards for detox. Clays fall between chlorella and charcoal on the selective absorption scale, binding to some beneficial minerals and nutrients. However, clay prevents absorption of heavy metals, VOC, mycotoxins, and other biotoxins.

Fruit Pectin

You can find pectin in apple pulp, citrus fruit peels, quinces, cherries, plums, and other fruits and vegetables. Fruit pectin is a weak binder that prevents heavy metals, mycotoxins, herbicide, and pesticide absorption. Despite its relative weakness, fruit pectin has anti-inflammatory benefits, and its high fiber content is an excellent food source for gut bacteria.

Humic and Fulvic Acids

Humic and fulvic acids are negatively charged atoms that attract positively charged mineral particles. Decomposing organic matter creates humic and fulvic acids. These compounds are excellent for removing heavy metals, environmental toxins, and even glyphosate. Perhaps the best news is that humic and fulvic acids are gentle enough to be taken with food.

PREVENTING TOXIC BEHAVIORS

I frequently tell patients that preventing or limiting their toxic product exposure is only half the battle. They must also prevent and limit the unhealthy behaviors contributing to their weight problems. Confronting our toxic food behaviors and habits requires an honest inventory. In time, many of my patients come to the uncomfortable realization that they're perpetuating the harmful behavior.

So, in this section, I've laid out some concrete steps you can take to be better and unlearn these health-destroying habits. However, I think the best way to start talking about preventing toxic food behavior is to look at the example of my patient Renata.

Renata's Story

Renata is a tough cookie.

She uses an iron will to power her way through life. Despite being mildly obese and sedentary most of her life, Renata took up martial arts at age fifty-one. Three years later, she'd earned a brown belt. Renata also raised three kids, worked part-time in a dentist's office, and volunteered at a local hospital. She survived a malignant melanoma diagnosis in her thirties and nursed her husband back to health after he had a stroke.

Though Renata is a tough cookie, she's not tough around cookies. Indeed, she goes weak in the knees at the sight of chocolate chips, Oreos, and snickerdoodles. She confided that she once devoured an entire box. Unfortunately, while Renata loves cookies, they don't love her back. Her cookie habit was adding thousands of extra calories every month.

Negotiation was Renata's default strategy for dealing with her cookie habit. "I'd sit there and tell myself, 'I'll just have a taste, maybe one or two mini cookies.'" The problem is that Renata never has one or two mini cookies and stops. Instead, those one or two cookies always became ten to twelve cookies. It happens every time she tries to negotiate portion size. Finally, in an honest moment in my office, Renata confided that she'd never been able to control herself around cookies.

"So, why do you keep negotiating with them?" I asked. "You have a long history of overeating cookies. What makes you think you're going to break this habit now?"

While it may appear that I was being negative with Renata, I was merely pointing out something she already knew. So, together, we decided it would be best for Renata to go cold turkey and give up cookies. And believe it or not, after sixty-four years of loving cookies, she did just that.

You might wonder how Renata could give up the one food that had been her siren song. It's not that Renata can't have cookies. She can have anything she wants. But Renata knows that the life she envisions will remain out of reach without a clean cookie break. So, she made the adult decision to exclude cookies from her diet because they didn't work for her control, and her history told us that they were a food she constantly abused. So, Renata used a strategy to prevent cookies from interfering with her weight-loss goals.

Renata's only concern was that she was removing a favorite food from her life. People who exclude certain foods or food groups may feel deprived—it's the number-one reason for failure across most weight-loss programs. So, I suggested that Renata find a substitute for her trigger food. A colleague asks every patient the same simple question about foods to include or exclude from their diet: "Does it satisfy or stimulate?" If you eat food that triggers cravings and makes you want more, then you know that's not a good choice.

Can pattern theory prevent toxic food behavior?

Have you ever heard of pattern theory?

The term was first introduced in the 1970s by Swedish statistician Ulf Grenander as a name for a field of applied mathematics. In lay terms, it's the analysis of the patterns the world generates in any modality, with all their naturally occurring complexity and ambiguity. The goal is to reconstruct the processes, objects, and events that produced those patterns. So, why am I talking about pattern theory in a book about obesity?

Like any other modality, eating behavior follows predictable patterns. Look at your own life. Do you overeat the same foods? Do you skip meals? Do you eat late at night? Do you eat when you're depressed or bored? Most people's eating behavior follows predictable patterns from childhood, when eating habits form, and track well into adulthood.

Exploring our eating patterns helps us understand when, where, why, and how we get into trouble. New York–based health psychologist Dr. Stephen Gullo refers to this unique eating pattern as an "eating print." Just as you have a unique fingerprint, you also have your unique eating print. Says Dr. Gullo, "Your eating print is a dynamic pattern of foods, behaviors, and situations that trigger you to lose control of your eating. A repetitive pattern forms a predictable mosaic of your food weaknesses and eating behaviors. Recognizing your eating print is one of the best weight control strategies."[11]

Strategy above All

In the last section, Identify, I examine the importance of identifying the eating habits that undermine your weight-loss efforts. But the way to prevent these behaviors isn't through willpower. Instead, it takes strategy to keep toxic behaviors at bay.

And one of the best strategies to lose weight and keep it off is to change your thinking. Weight management isn't simply about changing your toxic exposures. It also requires a paradigm shift in thinking and behavior. It will not happen if you jump from one fad diet to another.

To be successful, be aware of the role that eating plays in your life and learn how to use positive thinking and behavioral coping strategies to manage your eating and weight. Here are some ideas for preventing toxic behaviors and thinking:

1. Never go into food situations very hungry. What would you think if I told you to eat something before dining at a fancy

restaurant? That advice must seem crazy. However, I can't tell you how many people will starve themselves all day in anticipation of a big meal. Skipping meals and snacks all but guarantees that you will overeat at dinner. So, I suggest you have a lean protein and fiber snack beforehand to keep dinner from becoming a bacchanal. I have a patient who likes to eat a single-serving cup of yogurt topped with seven or eight nuts and some apple slices before she leaves for a restaurant or orders takeout.

2. Keep a food diary. It helps make you accountable. However, don't just write down what you eat and drink. Also include any thoughts and feelings that come up. Also, keep track of your behaviors. Were you stressed or depressed? Did you eat when you weren't hungry?

3. Limit or forgo nighttime eating. Late-night eating affects our hunger levels, how we burn calories after eating, and how we store fat.

4. Do drink plenty of water. Water aids satiety by helping you feel fuller and less hungry.

5. Try distracting yourself. Deep breathing, texting, talking on the phone, exercising, and walking are healthy activities to try when you experience cravings.

6. Be mindful during meals. People eat more while watching TV, working, driving, or standing. When you sit down for a meal, you take time to enjoy your food and eat more slowly. Food stays in your stomach longer, helping you feel full after your meal. Sitting down to eat also helps you to manage your portion size and avoid extra calories.

7. Look for support to stay motivated and accountable. The behaviors of others often influence how we behave. Knowing you have a group of like-minded friends cheering from the sidelines is a great way to stay focused, motivated, and accountable. Shared experiences allow us to be part of something greater than ourselves.

8. Be gentle with yourself. Try not to beat yourself up when you fall off the wagon.

9. Use the bathroom scale mindfully. Scales don't keep people thin. Every person with weight issues owns a scale. Instead of obsessively checking your weight, consider weighing your thinking and behaviors.

E—Eliminate

I hope by now you're convinced that prevention is the best medicine, as the saying goes. However, we also know that hazardous chemicals and their residues exist in every person on this planet. Even if you manage to prevent some exposures and absorption, there's simply no way to avoid all of them. Your body's burden of toxic chemicals and pollutants has accumulated since you were in your mother's womb. Various toxins fill our homes, workspaces, and recreational areas. We spray our food with pesticides, make children's toys of synthetics and plastics, and wash our hair with carcinogen-containing shampoo. Moreover, no one regulates the sale of these products—no wonder we're all effectively walking landfills.

However, we're not helpless in the face of this onslaught. Our bodies have built-in mechanisms for eliminating toxins and other harmful substances, of which the liver is a prime example. It breaks them down, converting them into safer substances, eliminates them through bile, or repackages them into a safer, water-soluble form that the kidneys can excrete. The liver will even store toxins to protect the rest of the body.

The lungs are also an effective detox organ. For example, our body produces carbon dioxide when converting food to energy. We rid our bodies of it by breathing it out. The lungs also have cilia fibers that push out contaminants. So, if you breathe in foreign particles, and everything is functioning optimally, the cilia's mucus traps them, and you cough up or swallow the invader, and it goes away.

The liver, kidneys, and colon are the three organs that eliminate waste and harmful substances. Your colon, or large intestine, is like a self-cleaning oven that has evolved over hundreds of thousands of years. After your small intestine absorbs the nutrients you eat, your large intestine gets rid of whatever remains.

The liver also plays a crucial role in digestion and performs many other functions. One is filtering your blood to neutralize and help your body eliminate potentially harmful substances. Whether you eat it, absorb it through your skin, or inhale it, however something unwanted gets into your bloodstream, the liver will process it. Your kidneys also filter your blood, removing byproducts of digestion and other bodily processes by producing the urine that flushes them from your body. However, a toxin must be water-soluble for the kidneys to excrete it.

DEFINING DETOX

What does "detox" mean? Detox, short for detoxification, refers to abstaining from and ridding the body of unhealthy substances or toxins to improve one's health. Our bodies detoxify independently, all day, without outside assistance. Healthy people typically do not require additional detoxification help. A healthy liver filters 47 ounces of blood every minute. The liver plays the most significant role in cleansing the blood. A healthy liver not only filters toxins and unwanted byproducts from the blood but also pulls nutrients from it to deliver to the rest of the body. In addition, the liver breaks down waste into relatively harmless water-soluble substances that the kidneys can excrete. For instance, the liver metabolizes alcoholic beverages and the majority of medications. With such a workload, the liver prioritizes what it does first, and clearing toxic molecules is way down on the list.

So, it's no wonder our liver and body need help. What, if anything, can we do to help our bodies eliminate these harmful substances?

SHOULD I TEST FOR TOXINS?

Some patients ask if they can test for toxins. There are ways to test hair, blood, and urine for toxins. However, these tests are not always helpful and can be expensive. Since we know every person has toxins in them and that the tests are imperfect and costly, experts do not recommend routine testing. I agree with them. In rare cases, a medical professional may recommend testing, often following known exposure to a harmful chemical at work or elsewhere. For example, we test some people with dental work or metal implants. However, most people will not benefit from testing.

CAN DETOXIFICATION DO MORE HARM THAN GOOD?

Many companies advertise supplements, products, foods, and packages meant to remove toxins from your body. They have little to no scientific proof these products work, and they can be pretty expensive. Some detox programs have so few nutrients that people may not get what they need for health, growth, and the body to work correctly. Some are very low in calories, which, over time, can be harmful. One danger is rapid weight loss. With rapid weight loss, toxins stored in fat go into the blood. From there, they can affect other organs. Fasting or being constantly hungry causes stress. When the body is stressed, the stress hormone cortisol goes up. High cortisol levels increase appetite. Fasting or very low-calorie diets can be safe and helpful under medical supervision. Some detox programs say that side effects like fatigue, headaches, nausea, and anxiety are regular responses to toxins leaving the body. That's not true. These symptoms are most likely caused by not eating enough calories. Stress from detoxing may make eating problems, such as binging, worse.

In the previous section, we focus on binders, products that help prevent the body's absorption of toxic compounds. Many of the supplements listed below are both eliminators and binders. Before trying, please discuss supplements, detox products, and new diets with a doctor or qualified healthcare professional.

A Note about Zeolites and Other Therapies

While the author, Dr. Lonky, is a licensed, board-certified medical professional, the therapies listed below should not be considered as replacements for personalized medical care. It's crucial to consult with a qualified healthcare provider before attempting any of the therapeutic techniques described in this book.

The effectiveness of therapeutic approaches can vary widely from person to person, and there is no guarantee of specific outcomes. It's important to exercise caution and use your own judgment when implementing these therapies, taking into consideration your individual needs and circumstances.

If you are currently undergoing medical or psychological treatment, it is advisable to consult your healthcare provider or mental health professional before incorporating any new therapeutic techniques.

ZEOLITES

Zeolite is the only substance in the world to effectively eliminate a wide range of toxic molecules and substances from your body. Zeolites are taken orally, usually as a liquid, but are also available as powders or capsules. With hundreds of studies touting the benefits of one of these zeolites, clinoptilolite, this mineral has gained increasing notoriety for its natural ability to trap toxins, heavy metals, and environmental pollutants.

How does it work? The first way zeolites work is through their cationic exchange abilities, meaning that negatively charged zeolites attract positively charged particles. In nature, four exchangeable metals called cations—usually calcium, magnesium, sodium, and potassium—balance clinoptilolite's negative charge. These cations are loosely held in the clinoptilolite structure and are readily exchanged for other positively charged substances.

Clinoptilolite's 3-D lattice-like framework resembles a honeycomb and these "cages" within the honeycomb can be filled with ions. This zeolite is microporous, with holes or pores less than 2 nm in diameter. Zeolites' tiny pores allow them to absorb molecules and ions that are smaller than the size of the pore openings. Zeolites willingly exchange a weakly charged, large calcium ion from their cage-like structure for a smaller ion with a strong positive charge that tightly fits the space inside the cage, such as heavy metals (mercury, copper, nickel, and lead). Once inside the cages, these toxic heavy metals are no longer active in the body and are flushed out permanently, since clinoptilolite is water soluble. The zeolite-heavy metal complex winds up in the urine.

Cationic exchange works perfectly for particles small enough to fit inside the zeolite cage, but what happens if you have large positively charged molecules, such as those found in VOCs? The zeolite sandwiches those particles. Two or more negatively charged clinoptilolite plates stick to various points on the positively charged larger toxic compound and haul it off naturally through the body. So, clinoptilolite will remove VOCs such as benzene, toluene, and acetone, even though they're not technically "inside" the clinoptilolite cage. These plates also attach to various other positively charged organic compounds.

LOOK FOR A ZEOLITE WITH ZETA POTENTIAL

Zeta potential describes a particle's electrical potential. Electricity matters since charge strength is how we measure zeolite's effectiveness. Usually, when you look at the structure of zeolite crystals, there are a lot of empty spaces between the pore and channel intersections. These spaces are like gaps of air where a charge weakens. However, the charge can bridge the gap and connect if you reduce the distance between the points (by making it smaller).

Applying the concept of zeolites' zeta potential means the entire particle becomes charged, allowing it to attract heavy metals and VOCs. However, zeta potential only applies to zeolites in a colloidal suspension where the particle size and charge converge to create an electrical potential. Therefore, the particle size needs to be small enough to enter the bloodstream.

Clinoptilolite is the only zeolite with zeta potential. It's also the only zeolite used for medical purposes in animals and humans and has excellent safety and efficacy profiles. Given its effectiveness, clinoptilolite is the best product to add to your daily detoxification regimen. Of all the purported detox products, clinoptilolite is the only one that gets into the bloodstream, according to the data. In many ways, it's like a toxin magnet—when you take clinoptilolite, it travels through your body, trapping toxins in its "magnetized" honeycomb cages or between the sheets of zeolite. Since your body doesn't store zeolite, it just excretes it along with any bound toxins. In this way, zeolite is exceptionally effective at eliminating built-up toxins in your body.

CHELATION THERAPY

Chelation therapy is a medical treatment that involves the administration of chelating agents, which are substances that bind to and remove heavy metals or minerals from the body. All FDA-approved chelation products require a prescription and can only be used safely under the supervision of a healthcare practitioner. However, over-the-counter (OTC) chelation products are available that claim to provide health benefits, though these are not FDA-approved for treatment of specific medical conditions. It's best to avoid these products at all costs.

Medical chelation therapy can come in various forms, including:

1. **Intravenous (IV) chelation:** This is the most common form of chelation therapy. Chelating agents are administered directly into the bloodstream through a vein, usually in the arm. The therapy is typically performed in a clinical setting and can take several hours. EDTA (ethylene diamine tetra acetic acid) is one of the common chelating agents used in IV chelation therapy.

2. **Oral chelation:** Chelation therapy can also be administered orally, where chelating agents are taken as pills or capsules. However, oral chelation therapy is often considered less potent than IV chelation due to the possible constraints in the absorption of chelating agents through the digestive system.

3. **Topical chelation:** In some cases, chelating agents can be applied topically in cream or ointment forms. These are used for localized treatments, like removing heavy metals from the skin.

"Chelate" comes from the Greek root *chele*, "to claw." EDTA has a claw-like molecular structure that binds to heavy metals and other toxins. EDTA injections grab positively charged heavy metals and minerals such as lead, mercury, copper, iron, arsenic, aluminum, and calcium and remove them from the body.

Chelation therapy using EDTA is the medically accepted treatment for lead poisoning. Once injected into the bloodstream, EDTA traps lead and other metals, creating a compound that the body can expel through urine. The process generally takes one to three hours. Other heavy metal poisonings treated with chelation include mercury, arsenic, aluminum, chromium, cobalt, manganese, nickel, selenium, zinc, tin, and thallium. Chelating agents other than EDTA are also used to clear several of these substances from the bloodstream.

The FDA approved EDTA chelation therapy as a treatment for lead and heavy metal poisoning. It is additionally employed as an urgent remedy for hypercalcemia (excessively high calcium levels) and for managing ventricular arrhythmias (irregular heart rhythms) linked to digitalis toxicity. These are EDTA's only officially approved uses in the US.

There's some thought that EDTA may act as an antioxidant by removing metals that combine with LDL cholesterol, which can damage arteries. The theory is that eliminating metals that flow freely through arteries (such as copper or calcium) may slow down diseases such as atherosclerosis. However, research has not proved this theory. Indeed, many well-designed studies have found that EDTA is ineffective for treating heart disease.

Some experts believe EDTA could remove calcium from healthy bones, muscles, tissues, and diseased arteries. Many medical organizations, including the National Institutes of Health (NIH) and the American Medical Association (AMA), have publicly criticized and denounced the practice of EDTA chelation therapy for heart disease.[12]

Children, pregnant women, and people with heart or kidney failure should not have chelation therapy at any dose. Because there is concern that EDTA may deplete essential vitamins and minerals, EDTA chelation therapy is often given with essential nutrients (including calcium, B vitamins, vitamin C, and magnesium).

EDTA may decrease the effectiveness of warfarin—an oral anticoagulant commonly used to treat and prevent blood clots—increasing infection risk. In addition, EDTA can lower blood sugar, just like insulin. Together, they may dramatically reduce blood sugar levels.

OTHER MEANS OF DETOXIFICATION

When considering products and procedures that claim to help eliminate toxic compounds from the body, it's important to approach the topic with caution and be aware that some claims may lack scientific backing. The body has its natural detoxification mechanisms, primarily carried out by the liver, kidneys, and other organs.

However, certain interventions and substances are believed to support the body's natural detox processes. Remember to consult with a healthcare professional before trying new products or procedures, as individual health conditions can vary.

It's crucial to note that the scientific evidence supporting the effectiveness of these methods can vary, and some practices may have potential risks or side effects. Moreover, the body's natural detoxification processes are highly complex, and no one-size-fits-all approach exists. Before making significant changes to your diet or lifestyle, it's advisable to consult with a healthcare professional who can provide personalized guidance based on your health status and individual needs.

Here are some additional substances and practices that are commonly associated with supporting detoxification:

- **Glutathione** consists of three amino acids—glycine, cysteine, and glutamate. It's recognized as the ultimate antioxidant because, among its various functions, it helps counteract free radicals generated in the initial stages of liver metabolism— the first line of defense against toxins. Glutathione also aids in phase II liver reactions, which conjugate the activated intermediates produced during the first phase to make them water soluble for excretion by the kidneys.

- **B vitamins** help the liver and other organs convert and eliminate undesirable toxins from your body, playing a crucial role in proper detoxification. The B vitamins are also necessary to make glutathione. B6, B12, and folic acid supplementation can even reduce epigenetic damage caused by air pollution. The reduction may be due to their ability to increase glutathione production.

- **Turmeric** is an herb descended from the ginger spice family and is widely used throughout India, Asia, and Central America to enhance the color and flavor of certain foods. Turmeric's medicinal benefits are highly associated with its active ingredient, curcumin. Turmeric leaves and stems contain many bioactive compounds, including curcumin. While curcumin's antioxidant and anti-inflammatory properties draw much attention, our bodies don't absorb turmeric well, potentially compromising its many benefits. You get around this problem in two ways: Add a pinch of black pepper to increase turmeric's benefits and bioavailability. Or you can consume healthy fats such as avocados, nut butter, nuts, and fish to increase curcumin's bioavailability.

- **Milk thistle** seeds contain an active group of flavonoids called silymarin that may protect the liver and aid in detox. Silymarin may keep toxins from attaching to liver cells while holding free radicals in check. In addition, studies show that silymarin may help ease inflammation and promote cell repair. As a result, milk thistle may help people with chronic liver disease improve their reduced detoxification capability.

- You've probably heard it a hundred times, but **water** helps the body remove waste through sweating, urination, and bowel movements. However, the amount you need depends on your physical activity level, age, and overall health.

Though the body has built-in detoxification mechanisms, certain lifestyle choices can support these natural processes. Here are some habits that may help support the body's detoxification system:

- Don't smoke, and limit (or give up) alcohol consumption. Both tobacco smoke and alcohol affect organs, particularly those involved in detoxification. There's no health benefit to drinking alcohol or smoking.

- I'm sure you've heard it all before, but eating a nutrient-dense diet can help your body remove toxic compounds and other harmful substances. You should avoid, as much as possible, refined carbohydrates and added sugars. Instead, include anti-oxidant-rich foods such as berries and nuts (provided you don't overeat nuts), dark leafy green vegetables, complex carbohydrates such as quinoa or sweet potatoes, fresh herbs and spices such as cilantro, turmeric, and ginger. Cruciferous vegetables such as kale, broccoli, cauliflower, and Brussels sprouts are good for your liver. Some evidence suggests cilantro can reduce cadmium and other heavy metal levels. It's safe in moderate amounts.

- Oily fish is a beneficial nutrient source. However, some oily fish, such as tuna, are high in mercury. Similarly, a study in the journal *Environmental Research* found that eating even a single serving of freshwater fish per year could equal one month of drinking water with high levels of PFAS (perfluoroalkyl substances).[13] Even low doses of PFAS in drinking water may increase immune system suppression and introduce an endocrine-disrupting chemical. PFAS also appears to raise bad cholesterol and exacerbate reproductive problems.

- Did you know sleep can help clear toxic waste products accumulated in the brain? Indeed, one of the most exciting discoveries in the past decade is that the brain has a waste management system. The glymphatic system is a series of tubes that carry fresh fluid into the brain, mix the new liquid with the waste-filled fluid surrounding brain cells, and then flush the mix out of the brain and into the blood. This process occurs primarily during deep sleep. Also, microglia, specialized immune cells found in the central nervous system, including the brain, perform essential maintenance and cleaning processes while we sleep. Cerebrospinal fluid (CSF) washes in and out like waves during sleep, helping the brain eliminate accumulated metabolic "trash." This process is believed to become more efficient during sleep, as lowered neuronal activity results in decreased blood flow and pressure within the brain. As a result, CSF circulation increases to maintain proper pressure and facilitate waste clearance. As the blood leaves, the pressure in the brain also drops, so the cerebrospinal fluid needs to increase to maintain normal pressure in the absence of blood.[14]

COGNITIVE RESTRUCTURING

We all experience occasional negative thoughts, and they're normal despite being frequently labeled as wrong. Envision welcoming these thoughts instead of resisting or feeling guilty about them. This approach could potentially enhance psychological flexibility. To improve your well-being, consider embracing rather than penalizing negative thoughts and behaviors. They're meant to teach you, not defeat you, so their impact might diminish through acceptance.

But how can we do this? Fluctuating motivation makes habit change challenging. Here's one possible solution. Years ago, I discovered Acceptance and Commitment Therapy (ACT). It's one of the most powerful ways of helping people with weight problems overcome their ambivalence, resistance, or entrenched nutrition beliefs by focusing on taking mindful action that aligns with their values.[15]

Here are some ways to avoid the obesity thinking trap, courtesy of Acceptance and Commitment Therapy (ACT):

1. **Practice cognitive diffusion.** Many people who are obese have low self-esteem. They feel worthless and often suffer from depression and anxiety. They attach to negative thoughts even when doing so is unhelpful. But what if you could flip the script? Rather than seeing the world through distorted and unhelpful thinking, could you see these thoughts as separate entities? Scientists call this strategy "cognitive diffusion." The goal is to detach from unhelpful thoughts that stand in the way of better health. It's not the thoughts that are the problem; it's what you do with them. I have an idea: Instead of dwelling on a thought until it drives you to a cupcake or a bag of potato chips, try sitting with it. Forget about fighting, fleeing, or even eliminating the thought. Instead, see it for what it is—a thought. It has no power except the power you give it. You can't outrun it, so stop struggling. That's your superpower.[16]

2. **Expand and accept.** This step creates a space for unpleasant emotions, urges, thoughts, and sensations. While this might seem odd, the goal is to allow them to flow through you without resistance. You don't have to like or want these feelings. But allowing them to "just be" can help us avoid the trap of over-inflating or wasting energy on them, allowing us to move forward with less effort and angst.

3. **Connect with the present moment.** All behavior takes place in the present moment. You can't overeat a bag of potato chips tomorrow or demolish a breadbasket yesterday. When

it comes to engaging in life with our actions, the present moment is the only time when the behavior happens.

4. **Observe yourself.** Another one of the ACT pillars, the Observing Self, is just what the name implies. It's the part of ourselves that observes our thoughts, emotions, and other aspects of our inner world. The Observing Self helps us reflect on situations with self-awareness, illuminating our beliefs, patterns, behaviors, and emotions. Ideally, we engage the Observing Self to see our thoughts for what they are— just thoughts, which are just words—and to feel emotions for what they are—biochemical reactions to thoughts or a situation. Once we see a situation for what it is, we can better manage our thoughts, emotions, and actions.

5. **Clarify your values.** Clarifying values means getting in tune with what's important to you. Think of values as activities that give our lives meaning. Values are not goals in that we never "accomplish" a value. Instead, values are like a compass—they help us make choices based on the directions we want our lives to go. Values are individual beliefs that motivate us to act one way or another. They shape and guide our behavior. Connecting with our values can move our lives in meaningful directions, even when we're faced with challenges or painful experiences. Remember also that values are highly individualized. They are not based on what others expect of us or what we think we should be doing. We choose our values.

6. **Commit to action.** As the phrase implies, committed action is about setting goals—committing to them—and taking active steps toward achieving them. Below are some positive strategies to help with your commitment to action.

CONTROL YOUR HOME ENVIRONMENT

1. Eat while sitting down at the kitchen or dining room table. Do not eat while watching television, reading, cooking, talking on the phone, standing at the refrigerator, or working on the computer.

2. Keep tempting foods out of the house—you can't eat what's not there.

3. Keep tempting foods out of sight. If you see it, you'll be tempted to eat it.

4. Unless you are preparing a meal, stay out of the kitchen. After dinner, one of my patients puts a dog gate at the kitchen entrance.

5. Have healthy snacks, such as small pieces of fruit, cut-up vegetables, canned fruit, yogurt, low-fat string cheese, and nonfat cottage cheese, at your disposal.

CONTROL YOUR WORK ENVIRONMENT

1. Do not eat at your desk or keep tempting snacks at your desk.

2. Plan healthy snacks and bring them to work if you get hungry between meals.

3. During your breaks, go for a walk instead of eating.

4. If you work around food, plan the one item you will eat at mealtime.

5. Make it inconvenient to nibble on food by chewing gum, sucking on sugarless candy, drinking water, or having another low-calorie beverage.

6. Do not work through meals. Skipping meals slows down metabolism and may result in overeating at the next meal.

7. If there's food at a party or set out for a special occasion, pick the healthiest item, nibble on low-fat snacks brought from home, don't have everything offered, choose one option and take a small amount, or have only one beverage.

CONTROL YOUR MEALTIME ENVIRONMENT

1. Serve your plate of food at the stove or kitchen counter. Do not put the serving dishes on the table. If you put dishes on the table, remove them immediately after eating.

2. Fill half of your plate with vegetables, a quarter with lean protein, and a quarter with starch.

3. Use small plates, bowls, and glasses. A smaller portion will appear huge when it is in a little dish.

4. Politely refuse second helpings.

5. Limit food portions to one scoop/serving or less when fixing your plate.

DAILY FOOD MANAGEMENT

1. In between meals, replace eating with another non-food activity.

2. Wait twenty minutes before eating something you are craving.

3. Drink a large glass of water before eating.

4. Always have a big glass or bottle of water handy and drink throughout the day.

5. Avoid high-calorie add-ons such as cream with your coffee, butter, mayonnaise, and salad dressings.

6. I know it takes work, but consider writing down everything you eat. You'll be surprised by what you discover.

GROCERY SHOPPING

1. Food shopping when you're hungry or tired is akin to throwing a match to gasoline. As a result, you're more likely to make poor food decisions.

2. Shop from a list and avoid buying anything not on your list.

3. If you must have tempting foods, buy individual-sized packages and try to find a lower-calorie alternative.

4. Don't taste-test in the store.

5. Read food labels.

FOOD PREPARATION

1. If you tend to eat as you cook, try a blocking behavior such as chewing gum or having a Listerine Breath Strip while making meals. The breath strip has the added benefit of making food distasteful.

2. Use a quarter teaspoon if you have to taste-test your food.

3. Only make what you're going to eat, leaving yourself no chance for seconds.

4. If you have prepared more food than you need, portion it into individual containers and freeze or refrigerate it immediately. Even better, throw it out or pour dish soap on it. You'll thank me later.

5. Don't snack while cooking meals.

EATING

1. Eat slowly. Remember, it takes about twenty minutes for your stomach to signal your brain that it is full. Take your time, and make sure you're actually hungry before serving yourself more.

2. The ideal way to eat is to take a bite, put your utensils down, take a sip of water, cut your next bit, take a bite, put your utensils down, and so on.

3. Do not cut your food all at once. Cut as needed.

4. Take small bites and chew your food well.

5. Stop eating for a minute or two at least once during a meal or snack. Take breaks to reflect and have a conversation.

CLEANUP AND LEFTOVERS

1. Do not clean up if you are still hungry.

2. If possible, don't clean up immediately after eating. Leaving the dishes for a while gives your body time to send fullness signals, helping you make more mindful decisions about whether you need additional food.

3. Divide leftovers into smaller, reasonable portions before starting to clean up. This helps you avoid mindlessly consuming large quantities.

4. Stay hydrated while cleaning up by sipping water. Sometimes, our bodies can mistake thirst for hunger.

5. Allow some time to pass before going back for seconds. This gives your body a chance to recognize fullness, and you might find you don't need additional servings.

6. Listen to hunger cues. Before going for more, assess whether you're truly hungry or if you're eating out of habit or boredom.

7. Store leftovers out of sight. Once you've plated your meal, promptly store the remaining leftovers in the fridge. Having them out of sight can reduce the urge to eat more.

8. Brush your teeth right after your main meal. The minty freshness can act as a signal that eating time is over.

SOCIAL EATING

1. Do not arrive hungry. Eat something light before the meal.

2. Try to fill up on low-calorie foods, such as vegetables and fruit, and eat smaller portions of high-calorie foods.

3. Eat foods that you like, but choose small portions.

4. If you want seconds, wait at least twenty minutes after eating to see if you are actually still hungry or if your eyes are just bigger than your stomach.

5. Limit alcoholic beverages. Alcohol lowers inhibitions.

6. Do not skip other daily meals and snacks to save room for the special event. You're guaranteed to blow your calorie budget.

AT RESTAURANTS

1. Order à la carte rather than buffet style.

2. Order some vegetables or a salad for an appetizer instead of eating bread.

3. If you order a high-calorie dish, share it with someone.

4. Try an after-dinner mint with your coffee. If you do have dessert, share it with two or more people.

5. Don't overeat because you do not want to waste food. Instead, ask to take extra food home.

6. Ask the waiter to put half of your entree in a doggie bag before serving the meal.

7. Ask for salad dressing, gravy, or high-fat sauces on the side. Dip the tip of your fork in the dressing before each bite.

8. Avoid bread baskets. Ask your server to hold back the bread basket if bread products or baked goods are your issue. The biggest mistake people make is thinking they can stop after a single piece of bread or one roll.

AT A FRIEND'S HOUSE

1. Offer to bring a dish, appetizer, or dessert that works for you and your control.

2. Serve yourself when possible.

3. Stand or sit away from the snack table. Stay away from the kitchen or stay busy if you are near the food.

4. Limit your alcohol intake. Alcohol lowers inhibitions and might make you more likely to overindulge.

AT BUFFETS AND CAFETERIAS

1. Cover most of your plate with lettuce or vegetables. As a colleague says, "Vegetables should take up the most real estate on your plate."

2. Swap your dinner plate for a salad plate.

3. After eating, clear away your dishes before having coffee or tea.

ENTERTAINING AT HOME

1. Explore low-fat, low-cholesterol cookbooks.

2. Use single-serving foods like chicken breasts or hamburger patties.

3. Prepare low-calorie appetizers and desserts.

HOLIDAYS

1. Keep tempting foods out of sight.

2. Decorate the house without using food.

3. Have low-calorie beverages and foods on hand for guests.

4. Allow yourself one planned treat a day.

5. Don't skip meals to save up for the holiday feast. Instead, eat regular, planned meals.

MOVE

1. Prioritize exercise by making it a planned, daily activity.

2. When possible, walk to your destination.

3. Get an exercise buddy to hold you accountable.

4. Park at the edge of the parking lot, farthest from an entrance.

5. Always take the stairs or at least climb part of the way to your floor.

6. If you have a desk job, get up and stretch or walk around the office frequently.

7. Do something outside on the weekend, weather permitting, like hiking or bike riding.

HAVE A HEALTHY ATTITUDE

1. Make health your weight management priority. Have a goal to achieve a healthier you, not necessarily the lowest or ideal weight based on BMI or some other metric.

2. Be realistic. You didn't gain all your weight overnight, so don't expect immediate results.

3. Focus on forming good habits, not on dieting. Dieting usually lasts for a short time and rarely produces long-term success.

4. Think big picture. You are developing new healthy behaviors to keep for the next month, year, decade.

Navigating Toxic Compound Labels While Grocery Shopping: Your Guide to Informed Choices

When embarking on your food shopping journey, it's essential to be aware of toxic compounds that might be present in products. Here's a list of labels to keep in mind as you make your selections:

1. **Artificial Sweeteners:** Watch out for labels that include artificial sweeteners such as aspartame, saccharin, sucralose, and acesulfame potassium. These may have adverse health effects and can sometimes be found in "sugar-free" or "diet" products.

2. **Artificial Colors and Flavors:** Foods with added artificial colors and flavors can contain chemicals that may negatively affect health. Look for labels that mention "artificial colors" or "artificial flavors."

3. **Preservatives:** Ingredients like BHA (butylated hydroxyanisole), BHT (butylated hydroxytoluene), and TBHQ (tert-butylhydroquinone) are synthetic preservatives that are often used to extend shelf life but could pose health risks in large quantities.

4. **Partially Hydrogenated Oils:** Products containing partially hydrogenated oils are likely to have trans fats, which can raise LDL cholesterol levels and increase the risk of heart disease. Look for this label and avoid products with these oils.

5. **High-Fructose Corn Syrup (HFCS):** This sweetener is linked to obesity, diabetes, and other health issues. Be cautious of products that list high-fructose corn syrup or HFCS in their ingredients.

6. **Monosodium Glutamate (MSG):** MSG is a flavor enhancer that can cause adverse reactions in some individuals. Foods that contain MSG should be cautiously approached.

7. **Sodium Nitrite and Nitrate:** Commonly utilized as additives in processed meats, sodium nitrate, similar to sodium nitrite, can change into nitrosamine in the body when exposed to extreme heat or a highly acidic environment. Nitrosamine is a known carcinogen. Look for products that are free from sodium nitrite and nitrate.

continued

8. **Genetically Modified Organisms (GMOs):** Labels indicating that a product contains genetically modified organisms (GMOs) can help you make informed choices about the potential environmental and health impacts.

9. **Pesticide Residues:** While not directly labeled, choosing organic products can help you avoid foods with high pesticide residues, which can be harmful over time.

10. **BPA-Free:** In relation to packaging, look for labels indicating that a product is "BPA-free." Bisphenol A (BPA) is a chemical in some plastics that can leach into food.

11. **Certified Organic:** Opting for products with an "organic" label can reduce exposure to synthetic pesticides, herbicides, and other potentially harmful chemicals.

12. **Non-GMO Project Verified:** The Non-GMO Project Verified label indicates that a product has undergone testing to confirm its non-genetically modified status.

Being mindful of these labels and the potentially toxic compounds they highlight can empower you to make healthier choices while navigating the grocery aisles. Remember that reading ingredient lists and understanding labels can contribute to a safer and more conscious approach to food shopping.

Talley's Take: Jane's Story—A Medical Mystery and the Healing Power of AIPE

Jane was exhausted, and every muscle in her body was in knots. As a competitive bodybuilder, runner, part-time fitness model, and one of Hollywood's most sought-after character actresses, Jane typically put in twelve- to sixteen-hour days, six or seven days a week, so exhaustion and muscle soreness were constant companions.

So, after one especially grueling twelve-hour day on the set of a hit show where she enjoys a leading role, Jane didn't think anything of a little siesta on the couch in her dressing room trailer.

When she woke ninety minutes later, Jane's head was throbbing. She stood up and nearly toppled over. "The room was spinning. It was like a severe case of vertigo, and my head was pounding." Jane grabbed a few Tylenol and lay down. In time, the headache subsided.

At first, Jane just chalked the whole thing up to fatigue and the long days that didn't allow much downtime. However, after she experienced a second debilitating headache, accompanied by tinnitus (ringing in the ear) and dry, bloodshot eyes, Jane called her doctor, who recommended a full workup. But Jane had an important work trip coming up and so she told her doctor the earliest she could come in was two or three weeks later. The doctor advised Jane to get to his office as quickly as possible. "I promise, doc," she said. "Just give me a few weeks, and I'll be there, no problem."

It took two months for Jane to make it to her doctor's office. In the interim, her situation had gone from bad to worse. As Jane sat on the examination table, pain—aching, burning, prickling pain—consumed every inch of her 5'7", 137-pound frame. Lesions and rashes marred her formerly unblemished complexion, while her left foot exhibited signs of swelling. She was tired to the point where getting out of bed had become a Herculean task, and her once taut, muscled frame had started to atrophy. Jane even confided that her hair was beginning to fall out.

The doctor was also at a loss. Any number of illnesses could explain this symptom collection. A complete workup failed to turn up anything conclusive, so Jane's doctor recommended she see a neurologist. He was also at a loss. It could be small fiber sensory neuropathy, or thyroid abnormalities, or adrenal fatigue, or mast cell problems, or fourth nerve palsy, or endocrine problems—Jane's symptoms fit many conditions. Fourth nerve palsy would explain the vision problems, but again, the tests were inconclusive, only deepening the mystery.

There was, however, one symptom that transcended all the others. Jane complained to her doctor about a "burning, vibrating, twitching feeling" under her skin. "Sometimes, it feels like something is crawling under my skin," she told her neurologist. This pain alarmed Jane since it was unlike anything she had ever experienced and was difficult to explain to her doctor.

As a peak performance athlete, Jane came to me looking for help creating an eating plan to maximize her training and give her more energy. After Jane described how she felt, I realized we may have missed the most critical symptoms in looking for the most obvious culprits.

Jane had undergone several contrast MRIs two years earlier before two micro lumbar discectomies. During the most recent procedure, doctors removed small sections of intervertebral discs that were pressing on her nerves and causing debilitating pain. The MRIs and Jane's collection of symptoms led me to suspect gadolinium toxicity.

Gadolinium, a heavy metal used as a contrast agent, improves the visibility of body parts with abundant blood flow (such as the spine or tumors) on MRI scans, and is administered to approximately 30 million people annually.

Since gadolinium (Gd) is a heavy metal, it's highly toxic to humans. However, all MRI contrast agents include a chelating agent that binds to gadolinium to prevent toxicity. We know that gadolinium accumulates in different body parts, including the bones, brain, and kidneys. In 2015, the FDA issued a safety announcement explaining that it would investigate the risk of gadolinium-based contrast agent (GBCA) buildup in the brain. While the FDA didn't find enough scientific evidence proving that gadolinium accumulation in the brain can affect our health adversely, Jane's symptoms told a different story.

Blood, hair, and urine tests revealed what I'd already suspected. Jane's Gd level was 0.638 micrograms (mcg) excreted over a 24-hour period. Anything above 0.019 mcg is considered elevated. The severity of gadolinium toxicity varies from person to person. However, sufferers usually experience acute symptoms shortly after having a contrast MRI. These often go ignored or get chalked up to something else, and then chronic symptoms that are harder to ignore can appear, sometimes for years following. Jane didn't have the early acute symptoms that we could tie time-wise to her contrast MRIs, so it was hard initially to make the connection. Also, there's often very little difference between early and ongoing chronic symptoms.

I suggested Jane see Dr. Lonky, who could rid her body of gadolinium with micronized activated zeolite in just a few weeks. Gadolinium binds to zeolite and is subsequently eliminated through urine. Jane also took gabapentin, which helped blunt her debilitating nerve pain.

Jane's experience reminds me of the importance of pushing for answers and seeking out qualified healthcare professionals. It also demonstrates the power and efficacy of Dr. Lonky's AIPE program. Often, people who come to see doctors struggle to accept diagnoses. Jane did the opposite. She immediately accepted the gadolinium toxicity diagnosis. Together, we identified the source as the residue of multiple contrast MRIs, and we prevented any future episodes of gadolinium toxicity by eliminating future contrast MRIs. Should Jane need additional MRIs or a CT scan, there are now alternatives to gadolinium. One such option, manganese, shares many properties that make gadolinium an excellent imaging probe. Finally, we eliminated gadolinium from Jane's body using micronized activated zeolite.

Today, Jane is back to work and has resumed competitive bodybuilding. She started networking with other gadolinium toxicity patients and even started a support group for people affected by the toxic effects of gadolinium retained from contrast agents. "It's been a great way to support other sufferers while sharing ideas on how to deal with the symptoms," Jane told me. I also devised a diet and supplement regimen to keep Jane's nerves healthy, invigorate and rebuild her muscles, reduce pain, and address particular symptoms.

In time, I hope the allopathic medical community will recognize gadolinium toxicity as a legitimate medical condition. Until then, Jane and others must discover and understand that, for better or worse, their health is in their own hands. Whatever the health challenges, we all need to find support and credible information to help us make informed healing choices that support our overall well-being.

Author's Note

At birth, we're gifted with our remarkable bodies, finely crafted and efficient. In the early days of my medical career, I marveled at this precision and complexity and the human body's status as Earth's most intricate machine. During embryology class, I witnessed the incredible transformation from a perfectly created embryo into a potential mess of abnormalities, diseases, and altered growth. Despite these risks, the developmental process usually goes smoothly, leaving me studying and questioning the marvel of our bodies.

Obesity, like human biology, is intricate. My journey into understanding obesity began because I couldn't bear watching my patients suffer. Treating them with palliative solutions like CPAP machines was not enough; I had to comprehend the root causes of their weight issues.

My quest for answers led me through a maze of literature, scientific research, and consultations with colleagues, but I found many theories incomplete. The obesity epidemic isn't merely about overeating and lack of exercise; it's a multifaceted problem. Experts offered simple solutions to a complex issue, pointing fingers at sugars, fats, carbs, and eating times, and some even claimed the epidemic was a social construct.

As I delved deeper, I couldn't shake the feeling that something vital was missing. Why are babies gaining excessive weight? Why are our pets packing on the pounds? Why did the obesity rate in the US surge despite the supposed role of genetics, which takes thousands of generations to evolve significantly?

To unearth the answers, I turned to the basics, particularly the workings of fat cells. In *Outsmarting Obesity*, I distill the science enough to convey that fat cells are not just calorie storage; they play crucial metabolic and endocrine roles. Leptin, the first identified fat-secreted hormone, highlights the connection between fat cells and weight regulation. Research has since unveiled numerous fat cell–secreted hormones with roles in health and disease.

This book serves as an introductory course on the science and my discoveries regarding obesity, providing an intelligible and paradigm-shifting perspective. I've worked diligently to establish connections that might appear unconventional, shedding light on the underlying causes of overeating and inadequate exercise.

Over the past decade, I have explored the impact of external and internal environments on gene expression, particularly DNA methylation of CpG islands. Epigenetic changes emerged as the key to understanding obesity's growth.

I firmly believe that the heritability of epigenetic marks carries more weight than our actual genes in determining our obesity risk. Ancestral and direct exposure to environmental toxins, chemicals, and drugs increase our susceptibility to obesity and metabolic dysregulation. These exposures reprogram the germ line's epigenome, passing down disease risk through epigenetic transgenerational inheritance.

My understanding grew as I realized the frequency of epigenetic changes correlated with the proliferation of environmental chemicals. Our reliance on convenience products, often laden with endocrine-disrupting chemicals, puts us at risk. Despite technological advances, we continue subjecting ourselves to chemical experimentation, compromising our health.

Reflecting on my upbringing, I have come to realize how fortunate I was to grow up without the influence of these modern conveniences. Today, despite their potential health risks, we take non-stick cookware and stain-resistant fabrics for granted. Manufacturers' switch from one chemical to another doesn't mitigate the endocrine disruption these products cause.

Our convenience addiction perpetuates the use of these chemical-laden products, and we play a dangerous game with our health. Robert Louis Stevenson's words, "Sooner or later, everyone sits down to a banquet of consequences," resonate as we confront the fallout of our choices. It's crucial to reassess our reliance on convenience and acknowledge the potential long-term repercussions, recognizing that our well-being is intricately connected to daily decisions.

Despite our desire to find a magic solution for weight loss and maintenance, we continue to gain weight. It's ironic that as society advances, we grow unhealthier. This collective indifference to the issues at hand suggests that we may not be as evolved as we think.

Obesity, a topic often shrouded in stigma, now faces a new layer of complexity in 2023 with sociopolitical issues. Those who bring attention to the problem may be labeled as fat shamers. It's essential to distinguish between meanness and raising health awareness. While nobody should be bullied for their weight or food choices, promoting the idea that a BMI of 35 is as healthy as a BMI of 23 is an irresponsible form of denial.

In *Outsmarting Obesity*, I address obesity candidly, recognizing the need to identify the problem to outsmart it. This book aims to provide a starting point for a deeper understanding of the obesity epidemic and how the future depends on it.

—Stewart Lonky, MD

Additional Resources

RECOMMENDED BOOKS

1. *The Obesity Code: Unlocking the Secrets of Weight Loss* by Dr. Jason Fung

2. *Mindless Eating: Why We Eat More Than We Think* by Brian Wansink, PhD

3. *The End of Dieting: How to Live for Life* by Dr. Joel Fuhrman

4. *Food Rules: An Eater's Manual* by Michael Pollan

5. *The Obesity Epidemic: What Caused It? How Can We Stop It?* by Zoe Harcombe

6. *The Skinny Jeans Diet: Change Your Thinking, Change Your Eating, and Finally Fit Into Your Pants!* by Lyssa Weiss, RD

7. *The Noom Mindset* by Noom

8. *Sicker, Fatter, Poorer: The Urgent Threat of Hormone-Disrupting Chemicals to Our Health and Future . . . and What We Can Do about It* by Leonardo Trasande, MD

9. *The Thin Commandments Diet: The Ten No-Fail Strategies for Permanent Weight Loss* by Stephen Gullo, PhD

ONLINE RESOURCES

1. National Institute of Diabetes and Digestive and Kidney Diseases (niddk.nih.gov)

2. American Heart Association (heart.org)

3. Obesity Action Coalition (obesityaction.org)

4. Centers for Disease Control and Prevention (cdc.gov/obesity/index.html)

5. ConscienHealth (conscienhealth.org)

6. ObesityHelp (obesityhelp.com)

7. Environmental Working Group (ewg.org)

8. Life Extension Foundation (lifeextension.com)

PROFESSIONAL ORGANIZATIONS

1. American Society for Metabolic and Bariatric Surgery (asmbs.org)

2. The Obesity Society (obesity.org)

3. The European Association for the Study of Obesity (easo.org)

4. Obesity Medicine Association (obesitymedicine.org)

5. World Obesity Federation (worldobesity.org)

6. National Obesity Foundation (nationalobesityfoundation.org)

7. International Association for the Study of Obesity (iaso.org)

8. American Association of Clinical Endocrinology (aace.com)

9. American College of Sports Medicine (acsm.org)

COMPANIES

1. Precision Food Works (precisionfoodworks.com)—nutritional catering and nutritional analysis

2. Avini Health (avinihealth.com)—products designed to help eliminate and prevent the absorption of toxic molecules, support gut and microbiome health, and promote weight loss and management

3. Touchstone Essentials (thegoodinside.com)—high-quality, organic nutritional supplements and detox products

4. Waiora (buywaiora.com)—dietary supplements and wellness products, including those containing zeolite (clinoptilolite)

5. Codeage (codeage.com)—dietary and health supplements and nutritional products

6. Unicity (unicity.com)—dietary supplements, nutritional products, and skincare items

7. Zuma Nutrition (zumanutrition.com)—high-quality nutritional supplements and health education

8. Coseva (mycoseva.com)—Advanced Toxin and Contaminant Removal System (or Advanced TRS)

Remember to consult with healthcare professionals before starting any new diet, exercise, or supplement regimen to ensure they are suitable for your specific needs and circumstances.

Acknowledgments

First and foremost, I would like to acknowledge my deep appreciation for the contribution to this book by my friend and colleague Chris Talley. His recognition of the importance of this book allowed us to include the insights of a practitioner who advises not only elite athletes and entertainers but ordinary folks wanting to "be their best." Chris, your contribution to the book and my knowledge is much appreciated.

When I undertook this project seven years ago, I had decades of experience as a clinician and a thirst for understanding why we have been so unsuccessful in dealing with obesity. After scouring the literature and speaking with scientists and practitioners, I had a brain exploding with information and hypotheses, but no clue as to how to assemble them into a readable book. Without the assistance of my friend and guide David Nayor, this would have been just a smattering of facts and conclusions. I am indebted to David for his encouragement and guidance over this long period. This book is as much a product of his perseverance as mine.

A big shout-out to the team at Greenleaf Book Group in Austin. First, to Justin Branch, who read through my book proposal and saw the value of *Outsmarting Obesity*'s message and agreed to work with me to publish this book. Another big thank you to Tanya Hall, CEO at Greenleaf, who, together with Justin, gave this project the go-ahead.

I want to express my sincere gratitude to Lee Reed Zarnikau, my primary manuscript editor. Lee's editing approach brings out the best in people without being overly demanding. It was so rewarding to see how quickly she grasped every concept in the book and how she saw to it that the information stayed clear and honest—not an easy task when dealing with such a complex topic. Hats off to you, Lee, for putting up with me and steering me away from being repetitive, dull, or getting lost in scientific minutiae. Also, I want to thank Tenyia Lee for her expert copyediting and Brian Welch for his guidance of the rest of the team at Greenleaf. Their efforts are greatly appreciated.

Many others before me have studied the root causes of obesity, and a few of them have affected me, including Robert Lustig, MD, in his book *Fat Chance* and Michael Moss in his book *Salt, Sugar, Fat*. Dr. Jason Fung's *The Obesity Code* was another stimulus for me to keep asking questions. I thank these authors for their expertise.

Questions were the catalyst that fueled my determination to seek answers. As a UC San Diego teacher and a clinical professor at UCLA, I had many students and residents ask challenging questions. Still, I must acknowledge Tess Ventura, DNP, ANP-C, a nurse practitioner, who got me thinking more and more about obesity and why we had so many problems managing these patients in a critical care setting. She made me think, scour the literature, and ask questions that sometimes had elusive answers. For this, a tip of my hat to her.

I also need to thank my two mentors in my UC San Diego Medical Center fellowship program. The late Dr. Kenneth Moser and the late Dr. Gennaro Tisi each guided me through my training as a clinician and a researcher. Ken taught me to broaden my vistas in considering medical mysteries, and Gerry taught me to be methodical in my approach to research. Their influence on my career has been profound.

Even earlier in my training, as a medical student, I was introduced to the world of "bench" research by the late Dr. Harold Levey, a professor of physiology, who taught me how to be thoughtful, honest, and meticulous in my work in the laboratory, and who gave me some of the best research advice: "There are no bad results from experimentation, just bad conclusions." This has allowed me to be far more critical in researching and drawing conclusions from published research.

Last but certainly not least, I would like to acknowledge my wife and partner in life for more years than we wish to admit, for her devoted patience over all these years it took to get *Outsmarting Obesity* from idea to finished product. Marilyn, thank you for letting me pursue this project, even when it took time away from us. Ditto for my children and grandchildren, who got used to me disappearing into my study or talking on Zoom, even on our vacations. I love you all for your understanding.

Notes

INTRODUCTION

1. John F. Kennedy, "The Soft American," *Sports Illustrated*, December 1960, http://theleanberets.com/wp-content/uploads/2020/02/1960 -JFK-The-Soft-American-SI-VAULT.pdf.

2. Nathan Yau, "The Changing American Diet," FlowingData, accessed October 18, 2023, https://flowingdata.com/2016/05/17/ the-changing-american-diet/.

3. Ramish Cheema, "5 Most Obese Developed Countries in the World," Insider Monkey, April 25, 2023, https://www.insider monkey.com/blog/5-most-obese-developed-countries-in -the-world-1141007/5/.

4. Dan Halpern, "Dr. Do-Gooder," *New York Magazine*, April 11, 2019, https://nymag.com/health/features/25642/.

5. Sharon Begley, "Why Chemicals Called Obesogens May Make You Fat," *Newsweek*, March 14, 2010, https://www.newsweek.com/ why-chemicals-called-obesogens-may-make-you-fat-79445.

6. Kevin D. Hall and Scott Kahan, "Maintenance of Lost Weight and Long-Term Management of Obesity," *Medical Clinics of North America* 102, no. 1 (January 1, 2018): 183–97, https://doi.org/10.1016/j.mcna.2017.08.012.

CHAPTER 1

1. UWA Film Society, "READ: Woody Allen's 1971 Short Story 'Notes from the Overfed,'" February 26, 2015, https://uwafilm society.wordpress.com/2015/02/26/read-woody-allens-1971 -short-story-notes-from-the-overfed/.

2. Guardian Staff, "1968: The Year That Changed History," *Guardian*, January 17, 2008, https://www.theguardian.com/observer/gallery/2008/jan/17/1.

3. Eleanor Beardsley, "In France, the Protests of May 1968 Reverberate Today — and Still Divide the French," NPR, May 29, 2018, https://www.npr.org/sections/parallels/2018/05/29/613671633/in-france -the-protests-of-may-1968-reverberate-today-and-still-divide-the -french.

4. Cynthia Ogden and Margaret Carroll, "Prevalence of Obesity Among Children and Adolescents: United States, Trends 1963– 1965 Through 2007–2008," Centers for Disease Control and Prevention, accessed December 4, 2023, https://www.cdc.gov/nchs/data/hestat/obesity_child_07_08/obesity_child_07_08.htm.

5. World Health Organization, "Noncommunicable Diseases," September 16, 2023, https://www.who.int/news-room/fact-sheets/detail/noncommunicable-diseases.

6. IMARC Group, "United States Weight Management Market: Industry Trends, Share, Size, Growth, Opportunity and Forecast 2023–2028," accessed October 21, 2023, https://www.imarcgroup.com/united-states-weight-management-market#:~:text=Market %20Overview%3A,6.13%25%20during%202023%2D2028.

7. United States Department of Labor – Employee Benefits
    Security Administration, "FAQ on HIPAA Portability and
    Nondiscrimination Requirements for Workers," accessed October
    29, 2023, https://www.dol.gov/sites/dolgov/files/ebsa/about-ebsa/
    our-activities/resource-center/faqs/hipaa-consumer.pdf.

8. Paul F. Campos, "Our Imaginary Weight Problem," (opinion) *New
    York Times*, January 3, 2013, https://www.nytimes.com/2013/01/03/
    opinion/our-imaginary-weight-problem.html?_r=0.

9. Julia Hartley Brewer, "If Your Child Is Fat Then You Are a Bad
    Parent," *Telegraph*, November 10, 2015, https://www.telegraph
    .co.uk/news/health/11985974/If-your-child-is-fat-then-you-are-a
    -bad-parent.html.

10. Medical Daily, "Obesity In America: 94% Of Americans Blame
    Fat People For Being Obese, So Why Is It Still A Problem?,"
    January 23, 2014, https://www.medicaldaily.com/obesity-america
    -94-americans-blame-fat-people-being-obese-so-why-it-still
    -problem-267684.

11. Paul Taylor, Cary Funk, and Peyton Craighill, "Americans See
    Weight Problems Everywhere But In the Mirror," Pew Research
    Center, April 11, 2006, https://www.pewresearch.org/wp-content/
    uploads/sites/3/2010/10/Obesity.pdf.

12. Christopher Ingraham, "Nearly Half of America's Overweight
    People Don't Realize They're Overweight," *Washington Post*,
    December 1, 2016, https://www.washingtonpost.com/news/wonk/
    wp/2016/12/01/nearly-half-of-americas-overweight-people-dont
    -realize-theyre-overweight/.

13. Bruce Y. Lee, "More Evidence That Obesity Is A Global
    Catastrophe In Slow Motion," *Forbes*, April 7, 2016, https://www
    .forbes.com/sites/brucelee/2016/04/07/more-evidence-that-obesity
    -is-a-global-catastrophe-in-slow-motion/?sh=13bc0f0c44fe.

14. David Katz, "Dr. Katz: The Issues of Labeling Obesity as a Disease,"
    (column) *New Haven Register*, June 23, 2013, https://www
    .nhregister.com/connecticut/article/DR-KATZ-The-issues-of
    -labeling-obesity-as-a-11425794.php.

15. Carnegie Mellon University News, "Press Release: Recommended Calorie Information on Menus Does Not Improve Consumer Choices, Carnegie Mellon Study Shows," July 18, 2013, https://www.cmu.edu/news/stories/archives/2013/july/july18_menulabeling.html.

16. Richard L. Atkinson, "Etiologies of Obesity," chap. 9, accessed October 21, 2023, https://biomedik.fkunissula.ac.id/sites/default/files/drupalbaru/files/bahan_ajar/Atkinson%20Etiologies%20of%20obesity%20%28dr.%20Minidian%29.pdf.

17. Association for Pet Obesity Prevention, "2018 Surveys & Data," accessed October 21, 2023, https://www.petobesityprevention.org/2018. This page contains the summaries of the *Veterinary Clinic: Pet Obesity Prevalence Survey* and the *Pet Owner: Weight Management, Nutrition, and Pet Food Survey*.

18. Yann C. Klimentidis et al., "Canaries in the Coal Mine: A Cross-Species Analysis of the Plurality of Obesity Epidemics," *Proceedings of the Royal Society B: Biological Sciences* 278, no. 1712 (June 7, 2011): 1626–32, https://doi.org/10.1098/rspb.2010.1890.

19. Janardhan Mydam et al., "The Effect of Maternal Race, Ethnicity, and Nativity on Macrosomia Among Infants Born in the United States," *Cureus* 15, no. 5 (May 23, 2023): e39391, https://doi.org/10.7759/cureus.39391.

20. n.a., "High BMI and Pregnancy Weight Gain with Alan Peaceman, MD," October 21, 2023, produced by Northwestern University Feinberg School of Medicine, podcast, LibSyn audio, 00:21:19, https://www.feinberg.northwestern.edu/research/podcast/high-bmi-and-pregnancy-weight-gain.html.

21. Kristen E. Boyle et al., "Mesenchymal Stem Cells From Infants Born to Obese Mothers Exhibit Greater Potential for Adipogenesis: The Healthy Start BabyBUMP Project," *Diabetes* 65, no. 3 (March 1, 2016): 647–59. https://doi.org/10.2337/db15-0849.

22. National Heart, Lung, and Blood Institute, "Balance Food and Activity," last modified February 13, 2013, https://www.nhlbi.nih.gov/health/educational/wecan/healthy-weight-basics/balance.htm.

23. Margaret Gough Courtney and Alyssa Carroll, "Sex Differences in Overweight and Obesity among Mexican Americans in the National Health and Nutrition Examination Survey: A Comparison of Measures," *SSM-Population Health 20* (December 2022): 101297, https://doi.org/10.1016/j.ssmph.2022.101297.

24. Nathan K. W. Colbert et al., "Perinatal Exposure to Low Levels of the Environmental Antiandrogen Vinclozolin Alters Sex-Differentiated Social Play and Sexual Behaviors in the Rat," *Environmental Health Perspectives* 113, no. 6 (June 2005): 700–707, https://doi.org/10.1289/ehp.7509.

25. Chris E. Talsness et al., "Components of Plastic: Experimental Studies in Animals and Relevance for Human Health," *Philosophical Transactions of the Royal Society B* 364, no. 1526 (July 27, 2009): 2079–96, https://doi.org/10.1098/rstb.2008.0281.

26. Michael K. Skinner et al., "Ancestral Dichlorodiphenyltrichloroethane (DDT) Exposure Promotes Epigenetic Transgenerational Inheritance of Obesity," *BMC Medicine* 11, no. 1 (October 23, 2013): https://doi.org/10.1186/1741-7015-11-228.

27. Begüm Harmancıoğlu and Seray Kabaran, "Maternal High Fat Diets: Impacts on Offspring Obesity and Epigenetic Hypothalamic Programming," *Frontiers in Genetics* 14 (May 11, 2023), https://doi.org/10.3389/fgene.2023.1158089.

28. Carl Zimmer, "The Famine Ended 70 Years Ago, but Dutch Genes Still Bear Scars," *New York Times,* January 31, 2018, https://www.nytimes.com/2018/01/31/science/dutch-famine-genes.html.

29. Wendee Holtcamp, "Obesogens: An Environmental Link to Obesity," *Environmental Health Perspectives* 120, no. 2 (February 1, 2012): a62–a68, https://doi.org/10.1289/ehp.120-a62.

30. Jamie Morgan, "OSU Study Links Light Exposure to Obesity in Mice," The Lantern, October 24, 2010, https://www.thelantern.com/2010/10/osu-study-links-light-exposure-to-obesity-in-mice/.

31. Nikhil V. Dhurandhar, "Infectobesity: Obesity of Infectious Origin," *Journal of Nutrition* 131, no. 10 (October 2001): 2794S–2797S, https://doi.org/10.1093/jn/131.10.2794s.

32. Hisashi Noma, Kazuo Hara, and Takashi Kadowaki, "Association of Adenovirus 36 Infection with Obesity and Metabolic Markers in Humans: A Meta-Analysis of Observational Studies," *PLOS One* 7, no. 7 (July 25, 2012): e42031, https://doi.org/10.1371/journal .pone.0042031.

33. Dorottya Zsálig et al., "A Review of the Relationship between Gut Microbiome and Obesity," *Applied Sciences* 13, no. 1 (January 2, 2023): 610, https://doi.org/10.3390/app13010610.

34. Jonathan C. K. Wells, *The Metabolic Ghetto: An Evolutionary Perspective on Nutrition, Power Relations and Chronic Disease* (Cambridge, UK: Cambridge University Press, 2016), 1–21.

35. Leo Tolstoy, "Book 15, Chapter 47," in *War and Peace*, trans. Constance Garnett (Chicago: University of Chicago Press, 2007).

36. Kristin Wartman, "What's Really Making Us Fat?" *Atlantic*, March 8, 2012, https://www.theatlantic.com/health/archive/2012/03/ whats-really-making-us-fat/254087/.

37. Helene A. Shugart, "Circumstantial Case: The Environmental Story of Obesity," in *Heavy: The Obesity Crisis in Cultural Context* (New York: Oxford Academic, 2016), 34–50, https://doi.org/10.1093/ acprof:oso/9780190210625.003.0003.

38. Douglas Main, "BPA Is Fine, If You Ignore Most Studies about It," *Newsweek*, March 19, 2016, https://www.newsweek.com/2015/ 03/13/bpa-fine-if-you-ignore-most-studies-about-it-311203.html.

CHAPTER 2

1. Peter Lattman, "The Origins of Justice Stewart's 'I Know It When I See It,'" *Wall Street Journal*, September 27, 2007, https://www.wsj .com/articles/BL-LB-4558.

2. Bruce Y. Lee et al., "A Systems Approach to Obesity," *Nutrition Reviews* 75, suppl 1 (January 1, 2017): 94–106, https://doi .org/10.1093/nutrit/nuw049.

3. John P. H. Wilding et al., "Once-Weekly Semaglutide in Adults with Overweight or Obesity," *New England Journal of Medicine* 384, no. 11 (February 10, 2021): 989–1002, https://doi.org/10.1056/ nejmoa2032183.

4. John P. H. Wilding et al., "Weight Regain and Cardiometabolic Effects after Withdrawal of Semaglutide: The STEP 1 Trial Extension," *Diabetes, Obesity and Metabolism* 24, no. 8 (April 19, 2022): 1553–64, https://doi.org/10.1111/dom.14725.

5. University of Virginia Health System, "Scientists Discover 14 Genes That Cause Obesity: Findings Could Decouple Overeating from Harmful Health Effects," ScienceDaily, October 21, 2021, https://www.sciencedaily.com/releases/2021/10/211001100432.htm.

6. Hélène Huvenne et al., "Rare Genetic Forms of Obesity: Clinical Approach and Current Treatments in 2016," *Obesity Facts* 9, no. 3 (June 1, 2016): 158–73, https://doi.org/10.1159/000445061.

7. Michael W. Schwartz et al., "Obesity Pathogenesis: An Endocrine Society Scientific Statement," *Endocrine Reviews* 38, no. 4 (August 1, 2017): 267–96, https://doi.org/10.1210/er.2017-00111.

8. Jean Vague, "A Determinant Factor of the Forms of Obesity," *Obesity Research* 4, no. 2 (March 1, 1996): 201–3, https://doi .org/10.1002/j.1550-8528.1996.tb00535.x.

9. Marie Pigeyre et al., "Recent Progress in Genetics, Epigenetics and Metagenomics Unveils the Pathophysiology of Human Obesity," *Clinical Science* 130, no. 12 (June 1, 2016): 943–86, https://doi .org/10.1042/cs20160136.

10. Vidhu V. Thaker, "Genetic and Epigenetic Causes of Obesity," PubMed Central (PMC), January 1, 2017, https://www.ncbi.nlm .nih.gov/pmc/articles/PMC6226269/.

11. Obesity Medicine Association, "Obesity Algorithm," 2019, https:// obesitymedicine.org/wp-content/uploads/2019/05/Obesity -Algorithm-2019.pdf.

12. Eduardo Faerstein and Warren Winkelstein, "Adolphe Quetelet: Statistician and More," *Epidemiology* 23, no. 5 (September 1, 2012): 762–63, https://doi.org/10.1097/ede.0b013e318261c86f.

13. Obesity Medicine Association, "What Is Obesity?," accessed October 29, 2023, https://obesitymedicine.org/what-is-obesity/.

14. E. Rudin et al., "Obesity," in *Encyclopedia of Gerontology* 2nd ed. (St. Louis, Elsevier EBooks: 2007), 277–82, https://doi.org/10.1016/ b0-12-370870-2/00140-2.

15. Society for Endocrinology, "Adipose Tissue, You and Your Hormones," accessed October 29, 2023, https://www.yourhormones .info/glands/adipose-tissue/.

16. Rosanne Spector, "Timing of Stress-hormone Pulses Controls Weight Gain," Stanford Medicine News Center, April 3, 2018, https://med.stanford.edu/news/all-news/2018/04/timing-of-stress -hormone-pulses-controls-weight-gain.html.

17. Dympna Gallagher et al., "Adipose tissue distribution is different in type 2 diabetes," *American Journal of Clinical Nutrition* 89, no. 3 (March 2009): 807–814, https://doi.org/10.3945/ajcn.2008.26955.

18. Lindsey A. Muir et al., "Adipose Tissue Fibrosis, Hypertrophy, and Hyperplasia: Correlations with Diabetes in Human Obesity," *Obesity* 24, no. 3 (March 1, 2016): 597–605, https://doi.org/10.1002/ oby.21377.

19. National Institutes of Health – News and Events – Research Matters, "Fat Tissue Can Communicate with Other Organs," March 7, 2017, https://www.nih.gov/news-events/nih-research-matters/ fat-tissue-can-communicate-other-organs.

20. Hye Jeong Kim et al., "Effect of Diabetes on Exosomal MiRNA Profile in Patients with Obesity," *BMJ Open Diabetes Research & Care* 8, no. 1 (September 1, 2020): e001403, https://doi.org/ 10.1136/bmjdrc-2020-001403.

21. Annette Haworth, Howard E. Savage, and Nicholas Lench, "Chapter 4 – Diagnostic Genomics and Clinical Bioinformatics," *Medical and Health Genomics* (June 10, 2016): 37–50, https://doi .org/10.1016/b978-0-12-420196-5.00004-6.

22. Marcelo A. Mori et al., "Role of MicroRNA Processing in Adipose Tissue in Stress Defense and Longevity," *Cell Metabolism* 16, no. 3 (September 5, 2012): 336–47, https://doi.org/10.1016/ j.cmet.2012.07.017.

23. Gyongyi Szabo and Shashi Bala, "MicroRNAs in Liver Disease," *Nature Reviews Gastroenterology & Hepatology* 10, no. 9 (May 21, 2013): 542–52, https://doi.org/10.1038/nrgastro.2013.87.

24. Vicente Javier Clemente-Suárez et al., "The Role of Adipokines in Health and Disease," *Biomedicines* 11, no. 5 (April 27, 2023): 1290, https://doi.org/10.3390/biomedicines11051290.

25. Andreu Palou, Catalina Amadora Pomar, and Ana Rodríguez, "Leptin as a Key Regulator of the Adipose Organ," *Reviews in Endocrine and Metabolic Disorders* 23, no. 1 (February 1, 2022): 13–30, https://doi.org/10.1007/s11154-021-09687-5.

26. Matthew Fasshauer and Matthias Bluhur, "The Role of Adipokines in Health and Disease," *Biomedicines* 11, no. 5 (April 27, 2023): 1290, https://doi.org/10.3390/biomedicines11051290.

27. Katarzyna Zorena et al., "Adipokines and Obesity. Potential Link to Metabolic Disorders and Chronic Complications," *International Journal of Molecular Sciences* 21, no. 10 (May 18, 2020): 3570, https:// doi.org/10.3390/ijms21103570.

28. Deepesh Khanna et al., "Obesity: A Chronic Low-Grade Inflammation and Its Markers," *Cureus* 14, no. 2 (February 1, 2022): e22711, https://doi.org/10.7759/cureus.22711.

29. Mohammed S. Ellulu et al., "Obesity and Inflammation: The Linking Mechanism and the Complications," *Archives of Medical Science* 13, no. 4 (June 8, 2017): 851–63, https://doi.org/10.5114/ aoms.2016.58928.

30. Ellulu et al., "Obesity and Inflammation," 851–63.

31. *Mosby's Dictionary of Medicine, Nursing & Health Professions* (St. Louis: Elsevier EBooks, 2021), https://books.google.com/books?id=aW0zkZl0JgQC&printsec=frontcover#v=onepage&q&f=false

32. Andrew Pollack, "A.M.A. Recognizes Obesity as a Disease," *New York Times*, June 20, 2013, https://www.nytimes.com/2013/06/19/business/ama-recognizes-obesity-as-a-disease.html.

33. Hélène Huvenne et al. "Rare Genetic Forms of Obesity: Clinical Approach and Current Treatments in 2016," *Obesity Facts* 9, no. 3 (June 1, 2016): 158–73, https://doi.org/10.1159/000445061.

CHAPTER 3

1. Ben Shapiro, "Why Can't We Talk About America's Obesity Crisis? With Bill Maher," YouTube, May 11, 2022, video, 4:52 (transcript available), https://www.youtube.com/watch?v=Z-VBWIcOrl4.

2. Anna Tingley, "James Corden Responds to Bill Maher's Fat-Shaming Comments," *Variety*, September 13, 2019, https://variety.com/2019/tv/news/james-corden-responds-to-bill-mahers-fat-shaming-comments-1203335512/.

3. Blanca Herrera, Sarah Keildson, and Cecilia M. Lindgren, "Genetics and Epigenetics of Obesity," *Maturitas* 69, no. 1 (May 1, 2011): 41–49, https://doi.org/10.1016/j.maturitas.2011.02.018.

4. Anna Justice et al., "Protein-coding Variants Implicate Novel Genes Related to Lipid Homeostasis Contributing to Body-Fat Distribution," *Nature Genetics* 51 (March 2019): 452–469, https://doi.org/10.1038/s41588-018-0334-2.

5. BBC News, "Fat Map: Largest Genetic Blueprint of Obesity Revealed," February 11, 2015, https://www.bbc.com/news/health-31372156.

6. Amit V. Khera et al., "Polygenic Prediction of Weight and Obesity Trajectories from Birth to Adulthood," *Cell* 177, no. 3 (April 18, 2019): 587-596.e9, https://doi.org/10.1016/j.cell.2019.03.028.

7. Mathias Rask-Andersen et al., "Genome-Wide Association Study of Body Fat Distribution Identifies Adiposity Loci and Sex-Specific Genetic Effects," *Nature Communications* 10, no. 1 (January 21, 2019), https://doi.org/10.1038/s41467-018-08000-4.

8. Pirro G. Hysi et al., "Metabolome Genome-Wide Association Study Identifies 74 Novel Genomic Regions Influencing Plasma Metabolites Levels," *Metabolites* 12, no. 1 (January 11, 2022): 61, https://doi.org/10.3390/metabo12010061.

9. Ruth J. F. Loos and Giles S. H. Yeo, "The Genetics of Obesity: From Discovery to Biology," *Nature Reviews Genetics* 23, no. 2 (September 23, 2021): 120–33, https://doi.org/10.1038/s41576-021-00414-z.

10. Zongyang Mou et al., "Human Obesity Associated with an Intronic SNP in the Brain-Derived Neurotrophic Factor Locus," *Cell Reports* 13, no. 6 (October 29, 2015): 1073–80, https://doi.org/10.1016/j.celrep.2015.09.065.

11. Øyvind Helgeland et al., "Characterization of the Genetic Architecture of Infant and Early Childhood Body Mass Index," *Nature Metabolism* 4, no. 3 (March 21, 2022): 344–58, https://doi.org/10.1038/s42255-022-00549-1.

12. I. Sadaf Farooqi and Stephen O'Rahilly, "The Genetics of Obesity in Humans," Endotext – NCBI Bookshelf, December 23, 2017, https://www.ncbi.nlm.nih.gov/books/NBK279064/.

13. Amit Khera et al., "Polygenic Prediction of Weight and Obesity Trajectories from Birth to Adulthood," *Cell* 177, no. 3 (April 18, 2019): 587-596.e9, https://doi.org/10.1016/j.cell.2019.03.028.

14. GIANT Consortium, "Largest Ever Genome-Wide Study Strengthens Genetic Link to Obesity," Broad Institute, February 11, 2015, https://www.broadinstitute.org/news/largest-ever-genome-wide-study-strengthens-genetic-link-obesity.

15. Zachary J. Ward et al., "Simulation of Growth Trajectories of Childhood Obesity into Adulthood," *New England Journal of Medicine* 377, no. 22 (November 24, 2017): 2145–53, https://doi.org/10.1056/nejmoa1703860.

CHAPTER 4

1. Blanca Herrera and Cecilia M. Lindgren, "The Genetics of Obesity," *Current Diabetes Reports* 10, no. 6 (October 8, 2010): 498–505, https://doi.org/10.1007/s11892-010-0153-z.

2. Mitch Leslie, "Fat? Thin? Molecular Switch May Turn Obesity on or Off," *Science*, January 28, 2016, https://www.science.org/content/article/fat-thin-molecular-switch-may-turn-obesity-or.

3. National Human Genome Research Institute, "Epigenomics Fact Sheet," National Institutes of Health, March 9, 2019, https://www.genome.gov/about-genomics/fact-sheets/Epigenomics-Fact-Sheet.

4. Ethan Watters, "DNA Is Not Destiny: The New Science of Epigenetics," *Discover Magazine*, October 17, 2019, https://www.discovermagazine.com/the-sciences/dna-is-not-destiny-the-new-science-of-epigenetics.

5. Farooq Ahmed, "Epigenetics: Tales of Adversity," *Nature* 468, no. 7327 (December 23, 2010): S20, https://doi.org/10.1038/468s20a.

6. Luqi Shen et al., "Early-Life Exposure to Severe Famine Is Associated with Higher Methylation Level in the IGF2 Gene and Higher Total Cholesterol in Late Adulthood: The Genomic Research of the Chinese Famine (GRECF) Study," *Clinical Epigenetics* 11, no. 1 (June 10, 2019): 88, https://doi.org/10.1186/s13148-019-0676-3.

7. Maria Stella Campagna et al., "Epigenome-Wide Association Studies: Current Knowledge, Strategies and Recommendations," *Clinical Epigenetics* 13, no. 1 (December 1, 2021), https://doi.org/10.1186/s13148-021-01200-8.

8. Steve Taylor and Clare Parsons, "Are You What Your Mother Ate? The Agouti Mouse Study," ShortCutsTV, 2018, video, 14:00 (transcript available), https://search.alexanderstreet.com/preview/work/bibliographic_entity%7Cvideo_work%7C4009609.

9. Vasantha Padmanabhan, "The Agouti Mouse Model: An Epigenetic Biosensor for Nutritional and Environmental Alterations on the Fetal Epigenome," *Nutrition Reviews* 66 (August 1, 2008): S7–11, https://doi.org/10.1111/j.1753-4887.2008.00056.x.

10. Max Planck Institute of Immunobiology and Epigenetics – Press Releases – Research News, "Epigenetic Switch for Obesity," accessed October 29, 2023, https://www.ie-freiburg.mpg.de/obesity.

11. Ranjani Lakshminarasimhan and Gangning Liang, "The Role of DNA Methylation in Cancer," *Advances in Experimental Medicine and Biology* 945 Springer Nature (November 9, 2016), 151–72, https://doi.org/10.1007/978-3-319-43624-1_7.

12. Charlotte Ling and Tina Rönn, "Epigenetics in Human Obesity and Type 2 Diabetes," *Cell Metabolism* 29, no. 4 (May 7, 2019): 1028–44, https://doi.org/10.1016/j.cmet.2019.03.009.

13. Cajsa Davegårdh et al., "DNA Methylation in the Pathogenesis of Type 2 Diabetes in Humans," *Molecular Metabolism* 14 (February 7, 2018): 12–25, https://doi.org/10.1016/j.molmet.2018.01.022.

14. Tina Rönn et al., "A Six Months Exercise Intervention Influences the Genome-Wide DNA Methylation Pattern in Human Adipose Tissue," *PLOS Genetics* 9, no. 6 (June 27, 2013): e1003572, https://doi.org/10.1371/journal.pgen.1003572.

15. Joseph Kochmanski et al., "Neonatal Bloodspot DNA Methylation Patterns Are Associated with Childhood Weight Status in the Healthy Families Project," *Pediatric Research* 85, no. 6 (May 1, 2019): 848–55, https://doi.org/10.1038/s41390-018-0227-1.

16. Natalia S. Harasymowicz et al., "Intergenerational Transmission of Diet-Induced Obesity, Metabolic Imbalance, and Osteoarthritis in Mice," *Arthritis & Rheumatology* 72, no. 4 (April 1, 2020): 632–44, https://doi.org/10.1002/art.41147.

17. Mark Newman, "The Epigenetics of Obesity," Endocrine News, March 11, 2016, https://endocrinenews.endocrine.org/the-epigenetics-of-obesity/.

18. Ida Donkin et al., "Obesity and Bariatric Surgery Drive Epigenetic Variation of Spermatozoa in Humans." *Cell Metabolism* 23, no. 2 (February 9, 2016): 369–78, https://doi.org/10.1016/j.cmet.2015.11.004.

19. Adelheid Soubry et al., "Newborns of Obese Parents Have Altered DNA Methylation Patterns at Imprinted Genes," *International Journal of Obesity* 39, no. 4 (April 1, 2015): 650–57, https://doi.org/10.1038/ijo.2013.193.

20. Gauri Deb et al., "Green Tea-Induced Epigenetic Reactivation of Tissue Inhibitor of Matrix Metalloproteinase-3 Suppresses Prostate Cancer Progression through Histone-Modifying Enzymes," *Molecular Carcinogenesis* 58, no. 7 (July 1, 2019): 1194–1207, https://doi.org/10.1002/mc.23003.

CHAPTER 5

1. J. Völker, et al., "Adipogenic Activity of Chemicals Used in Plastic Consumer Products," *Environmental Science & Technology* 56, no. 4 (January 26, 2022): 2487–96, https://doi.org/10.1021/acs.est.1c06316.

2. Gang Liu et al., "Perfluoroalkyl Substances and Changes in Body Weight and Resting Metabolic Rate in Response to Weight-Loss Diets: A Prospective Study," *PLOS Medicine* 15, no. 2 (February 13, 2018): e1002502, https://doi.org/10.1371/journal.pmed.1002502.

3. Matthew D. Anway and Michael K. Skinner, "Epigenetic Transgenerational Actions of Endocrine Disruptors," *Endocrinology* 147, no. 6 (June 1, 2006): s43–49, https://doi.org/10.1210/en.2005-1058.

4. Mohan Manikkam et al., "Plastics Derived Endocrine Disruptors (BPA, DEHP and DBP) Induce Epigenetic Transgenerational Inheritance of Obesity, Reproductive Disease and Sperm Epimutations," *PLOS One* 8, no. 1 (January 24, 2013): e55387, https://doi.org/10.1371/journal.pone.0055387.

5. Robert M. Sargis et al., "Environmental Endocrine Disruptors Promote Adipogenesis in the 3T3-L1 Cell Line through Glucocorticoid Receptor Activation," *Obesity* 18, no. 7 (July 1, 2010): 1283–88, https://doi.org/10.1038/oby.2009.419.

6. Felix Grün and Bruce Blumberg, "Environmental Obesogens: Organotins and Endocrine Disruption via Nuclear Receptor Signaling," *Endocrinology* 147, no. 6 suppl (June 1, 2006): S50-5, https://doi.org/10.1210/en.2005-1129.

7. Joyce M. Lee et al., "United States Dietary Trends Since 1800: Lack of Association Between Saturated Fatty Acid Consumption and Non-Communicable Diseases," *Frontiers in Nutrition* 8 (January 13, 2022), https://doi.org/10.3389/fnut.2021.748847.

8. Centers for Disease Control and Prevention, Publications – E-stats, "Prevalence of Overweight and Obesity Among Adults: United States, 2003–2004," accessed October 29, 2023, https://www.cdc .gov/nchs/data/hestat/overweight/overweight_adult_03.htm.

9. World Obesity Federation – News, "Economic Impact of Overweight and Obesity to Surpass $4 Trillion by 2035," accessed October 29, 2023, https://www.worldobesity.org/news/economic -impact-of-overweight-and-obesity-to-surpass-4-trillion-by-2035.

10. Robert H. Lustig et al., "Obesity I: Overview and Molecular and Biochemical Mechanisms," *Biochemical Pharmacology* 199 (May 1, 2022): 115012, https://doi.org/10.1016/j.bcp.2022.115012.

11. Philippe Grandjean et al., "Weight Loss Relapse Associated with Exposure to Perfluorinated Alkylate Substances," *Obesity* 31, no. 6 (April 17, 2023): 1686–96, https://doi.org/10.1002/oby.23755.

12. Jessica R. Shoaff et al., "Association of Exposure to Endocrine-Disrupting Chemicals during Adolescence with Attention-Deficit/ Hyperactivity Disorder–Related Behaviors," *JAMA Network Open* 3, no. 8 (August 28, 2020): e2015041, https://doi.org/10.1001/ jamanetworkopen.2020.15041.

13. Elizabeth Mendes, "The Study That Helped Spur the US Stop-Smoking Movement," American Cancer Society, January 9, 2014, https://www.cancer.org/research/acs-research-news/the-study -that-helped-spur-the-us-stop-smoking-movement.html.

14. Charles W. Schmidt, "TSCA 2.0: A New Era in Chemical Risk Management," *Environmental Health Perspectives* 124, no. 10 (October 1, 2016), https://doi.org/10.1289/ehp.124-a182.

15. United States Environmental Protection Agency – webpage for asbestos, "Asbestos Ban and Phase-Out Federal Register Notices," last modified July 3, 2023, https://www.epa.gov/asbestos/asbestos-ban-and-phase-out-federal-register-notices.

16. Teresa M. Attina et al., "Exposure to Endocrine-Disrupting Chemicals in the USA: A Population-Based Disease Burden and Cost Analysis," *Lancet* 4, no. 12 (December 1, 2016): 996–1003, https://doi.org/10.1016/s2213-8587(16)30275-3.

17. Kerri Arsenault, "Nine Questions for the Author: Leonardo Trasande, Author of *Sicker, Fatter, Poorer*," *Orion Magazine*, April 3, 2019. https://orionmagazine.org/2019/04/nine-questions-for-the-author-leonardo-trasande-author-of-sicker-fatter-poorer/.

18. California Department of Public Health – webpage for California Safe Cosmetics, "The Cosmetic Fragrance and Flavor Ingredient Right to Know Act of 2020 (SB 312): Compliance Information for Companies," accessed October 29, 2023, https://www.cdph.ca.gov/Programs/CCDPHP/DEODC/OHB/CSCP/Pages/SB312.aspx.

19. Leonardo Trasande, Teresa M. Attina, and Jan Blustein, "Association Between Urinary Bisphenol A Concentration and Obesity Prevalence in Children and Adolescents," *JAMA* 308, no. 11 (September 19, 2012): 1113, https://doi.org/10.1001/2012.jama.11461.

20. Elizabeth G. Radke et al., "Phthalate Exposure and Metabolic Effects: A Systematic Review of the Human Epidemiological Evidence," *Environment International* 132 (November 1, 2019): 104768, https://doi.org/10.1016/j.envint.2019.04.040.

21. Kelly J. Gauger et al., "Polychlorinated Biphenyls (PCBs) Exert Thyroid Hormone-Like Effects in the Fetal Rat Brain but Do Not Bind to Thyroid Hormone Receptors," *Environmental Health Perspectives* 112, no. 5 (April 1, 2004): 516–23, https://doi.org/10.1289/ehp.6672.

CHAPTER 6

1. Vanita Mehta et al., "Obstructive Sleep Apnea and Oxygen Therapy: A Systematic Review of the Literature and Meta-Analysis," *Journal of Clinical Sleep Medicine* 09, no. 03 (March 15, 2013): 271–79, https://doi.org/10.5664/jcsm.2500.

2. n. a., "Continuous or Nocturnal Oxygen Therapy in Hypoxemic Chronic Obstructive Lung Disease," *Annals of Internal Medicine* 93, no. 3 (September 1, 1980): 391, https://doi.org/10.7326/0003-4819-93-3-391.

3. "Continuous or Nocturnal Oxygen Therapy," 391.

4. Paul E. Peppard, Neil Ward, and Mary J. Morrell, "The Impact of Obesity on Oxygen Desaturation during Sleep-Disordered Breathing," *American Journal of Respiratory and Critical Care Medicine* 180, no. 8 (October 15, 2009): 788–93, https://doi.org/10.1164/rccm.200905-0773oc.

5. Shih-Chun Hsing et al., "Obese Patients Experience More Severe OSA Than Non-obese Patients," *Medicine*, 101, no. 41 (October 14, 2022): e31039, https://doi.org/10.1097/md.0000000000031039.

6. Nancy Kanagy, "Vascular Effects of Intermittent Hypoxia," *ILAR Journal* 50, no. 3 (January 1, 2009): 282–88, https://academic.oup.com/ilarjournal/article/50/3/282/770319.

7. Jianping Ye et al., "Hypoxia Is a Potential Risk Factor for Chronic Inflammation and Adiponectin Reduction in Adipose Tissue of Ob/Ob and Dietary Obese Mice," *American Journal of Physiology* 293, no. 4 (October 1, 2007): E1118–28, https://doi.org/10.1152/ajpendo.00435.2007.

8. Paul Trayhurn, "Hypoxia and Adipocyte Physiology: Implications for Adipose Tissue Dysfunction in Obesity," *Annual Review of Nutrition* 34, no. 1 (July 17, 2014): 207–36, https://doi.org/10.1146/annurev-nutr-071812-161156.

9. Sema Akgün, Tülay Köken, and Ahmet Kahraman, "Evaluation of Adiponectin and Leptin Levels and Oxidative Stress in Bipolar Disorder Patients with Metabolic Syndrome Treated by Valproic

Acid," *Journal of Psychopharmacology* 31, no. 11 (September 6, 2017): 1453–59, https://doi.org/10.1177/0269881117715608.

10. William C. Wheaton and Navdeep S. Chandel, "Hypoxia. 2. Hypoxia Regulates Cellular Metabolism," *American Journal of Physiology-Cell Physiology* 300, no. 3 (March 1, 2011): C385–93, https://doi.org/10.1152/ajpcell.00485.2010.

11. Ioannis G Lempesis et al., "Oxygenation of Adipose Tissue: A Human Perspective," *Acta Physiologica* 228, no. 1 (January 1, 2020), https://doi.org/10.1111/apha.13298.

12. Linda Rausch et al., "The Linkage between Breast Cancer, Hypoxia, and Adipose Tissue," *Frontiers in Oncology* 7 (September 25, 2017), https://doi.org/10.3389/fonc.2017.00211.

13. Jim Dryden, "Not All Obese People Develop Metabolic Problems Linked to Excess Weight," The Source – Washington University in St. Louis, January 13, 2016, https://source.wustl.edu/2015/01/not-all-obese-people-develop-metabolic-problems-linked-to-excess-weight/.

14. Elizabeth Williamson et al., "Factors Associated with COVID-19-Related Death Using OpenSAFELY," *Nature* 584, no. 7821 (July 8, 2020): 430–36, https://doi.org/10.1038/s41586-020-2521-4.

15. Yuefei Jin et al., "Endothelial Activation and Dysfunction in COVID-19: From Basic Mechanisms to Potential Therapeutic Approaches," *Signal Transduction and Targeted Therapy* 5, no. 1 (December 24, 2020), https://doi.org/10.1038/s41392-020-00454-7.

16. Giovanny J. Martínez-Colón et al., "SARS-CoV-2 Infection Drives an Inflammatory Response in Human Adipose Tissue through Infection of Adipocytes and Macrophages," *Science Translational Medicine* 14, no. 674 (September 22, 2022), https://doi.org/10.1126/scitranslmed.abm9151.

17. Jun Yang, Jiahui Hu, and Chunyan Zhu, "Obesity Aggravates COVID-19: A Systematic Review and Meta-analysis," *Journal of Medical Virology* 93, no. 1 (January 1, 2021): 257–61, https://doi.org/10.1002/jmv.26237.

18. Amiel A. Dror et al., "Pre-Infection 25-Hydroxyvitamin D3 Levels and Association with Severity of COVID-19 Illness," *PLOS One* 17, no. 2 (February 3, 2022): e0263069, https://doi.org/10.1371/journal .pone.0263069.

CHAPTER 7

1. Weijia Wang, "Beauty as the Symbol of Morality: A Twofold Duty in Kant's Theory of Taste," *Dialogue* 57, no. 4 (December 1, 2018): 853–75, https://doi.org/10.1017/s001221731800015x.

2. Sarah E. Jackson, Rebecca J. Beeken, and Jane Wardle, "Obesity, Perceived Weight Discrimination, and Psychological Well-Being in Older Adults in England," *Obesity* 23, no. 5 (May 1, 2015): 1105–11, https://doi.org/10.1002/oby.21052.

3. Rishi Caleyachetty et al., "Metabolically Healthy Obese and Incident Cardiovascular Disease Events among 3.5 Million Men and Women," *Journal of the American College of Cardiology* 70, no. 12 (September 19, 2017): 1429–37, https://doi.org/10.1016/ j.jacc.2017.07.763.

4. Ziyi Zhou et al., "Are People with Metabolically Healthy Obesity Really Healthy? A Prospective Cohort Study of 381,363 UK Biobank Participants," *Diabetologia* 64, no. 9 (June 10, 2021): 1963–72, https://doi.org/10.1007/s00125-021-05484-6.

5. Herculina S. Kruger et al., "The Metabolic Profiles of Metabolically Healthy Obese and Metabolically Unhealthy Obese South African Adults over 10 Years," *International Journal of Environmental Research and Public Health* 19, no. 9 (April 21, 2022): 5061, https:// doi.org/10.3390/ijerph19095061.

6. Meng Gao et al., "Metabolically Healthy Obesity, Transition to Unhealthy Metabolic Status, and Vascular Disease in Chinese Adults: A Cohort Study," *PLOS Medicine* 17, no. 10 (October 30, 2020): e1003351, https://doi.org/10.1371/journal.pmed.1003351.

7. Jiri Dvorak et al., "The Obesity Paradox in the Trauma Patient: Normal May Not Be Better," *World Journal of Surgery* 44, no. 6 (June 1, 2020): 1817–23, https://doi.org/10.1007/s00268-020-05398-1.

8. Maria Pina Dore et al., "Overweight: A Protective Factor against Comorbidity in the Elderly," *International Journal of Environmental Research and Public Health* 16, no. 19 (September 29, 2019): 3656, https://doi.org/10.3390/ijerph16193656.

9. Stamatina Iliodromiti et al., "The Impact of Confounding on the Associations of Different Adiposity Measures with the Incidence of Cardiovascular Disease: A Cohort Study of 296,535 Adults of White European Descent," *European Heart Journal* 39, no. 17 (May 1, 2018): 1514–20, https://doi.org/10.1093/eurheartj/ehy057.

10. Nicole O. Palmer et al., "Impact of Obesity on Male Fertility, Sperm Function and Molecular Composition," *Spermatogenesis* 2, no. 4 (October 1, 2012): 253–63, https://doi.org/10.4161/spmg.21362.

11. Pedro L. Valenzuela et al., "Joint Association of Physical Activity and Body Mass Index with Cardiovascular Risk: A Nationwide Population-Based Cross-Sectional Study," *European Journal of Preventive Cardiology* 29, no. 2 (January 2022): e50–e52, https://doi .org/10.1093/eurjpc/zwaa151.

12. Website of the National Association to Advance Fat Acceptance (NAAFA), accessed October 29, 2023, https://naafa.org/.

13. Public Health England, "Press Release: Campaign Launched to Help Public Get Healthy This Summer," GOV.UK, last modified September 14, 2021, https://www.gov.uk/government/news/ campaign-launched-to-help-public-get-healthy-this-summer.

14. Carl Baker, "Obesity Statistics," House of Commons Library, January 12, 2023, https://researchbriefings.files.parliament.uk/ documents/SN03336/SN03336.pdf.

CHAPTER 8

1. Bonnie Liebman, "Why Our Toxic Food Environment Matters," Center for Science in the Public Interest, last modified August 25, 2022, https://www.cspinet.org/article/why-our-toxic-food -environment-matters.

2. Thich Nhat Hanh, *How to Eat* (Berkeley: Parallax Press, 2014), 67.

3. Charles J. Courtemanche et al., "Can Changing Economic Factors Explain the Rise in Obesity?" *NBER Working Paper Series*, National Bureau of Economic Research, January 2015, https://www.nber.org/ system/files/working_papers/w20892/w20892.pdf.

4. Brian Wansink and Jeffery Sobal, "Mindless Eating," *Environment and Behavior* 39, no. 1 (January 1, 2007): 106–23, https://doi .org/10.1177/0013916506295573.

5. Drew DeSilver, "How America's Diet Has Changed over Time," Pew Research Center, December 13, 2016, https://www.pewresearch .org/short-reads/2016/12/13/whats-on-your-table-how-americas -diet-has-changed-over-the-decades/.

6. Robert B. Cialdini, *Influence: The Psychology of Persuasion* (New York: HarperCollins, 2006), 45.

7. Nina Hallowell, Shirlene Badger, and Julia Lawton, "Eating to Live or Living to Eat: The Meaning of Hunger Following Gastric Surgery," *SSM – Qualitative Research in Health* 1 (December 1, 2021): 100005, https://doi.org/10.1016/j.ssmqr.2021.100005.

8. G. R. Hervey, "The Effects of Lesions in the Hypothalamus in Parabiotic Rats," *The Journal of Physiology* 145, no. 2 (March 3, 1959): 336–52, https://doi.org/10.1113/jphysiol.1959.sp006145.

9. "Researchers Identify Genes That Directly Influence What We Eat," EurekAlert! (news release), July 22, 2023, https://www.eurekalert .org/news-releases/995549.

10. Karen A. Lillycrop and Graham C. Burdge, "The Effect of Nutrition during Early Life on the Epigenetic Regulation of Transcription and Implications for Human Diseases," *Lifestyle Genomics* 4, no. 5 (January 1, 2011): 248–60, https://doi.org/10.1159/000334857.

11. Richard D. Mattes, "Hunger and Thirst: Issues in Measurement and Prediction of Eating and Drinking," *Physiology & Behavior* 100, no. 1 (April 1, 2010): 22–32, https://doi.org/10.1016/j.physbeh .2009.12.026.

12. Lisa Martine Jenkins, "How NAFTA Changed the Way Americans and Mexicans Eat," Eater, September 19, 2018, https://www.eater .com/2018/9/19/17878946/nafta-mexico-america-trade -agreement-farming-diet.

13. Thomas J. Bollyky et al., "Pandemic Preparedness and COVID-19: An Exploratory Analysis of Infection and Fatality Rates, and Contextual Factors Associated with Preparedness in 177 Countries, from Jan 1, 2020, to Sept 30, 2021," *Lancet* 399, no. 10334 (April 1, 2022): 1489–1512, https://doi.org/10.1016/ s0140-6736(22)00172-6.

14. Tija Ragelienė and Alice Grønhøj, "The Influence of Peers' and Siblings' on Children's and Adolescents' Healthy Eating Behavior. A Systematic Literature Review," *Appetite* 148 (May 1, 2020): 104592, https://doi.org/10.1016/j.appet.2020.104592.

15. R. C. Kleseges et al., "Parental Influence on Food Selection in Young Children and Its Relationships to Childhood Obesity," *The American Journal of Clinical Nutrition* 53, no. 4 (April 1, 1991): 859–64, https://doi.org/10.1093/ajcn/53.4.859.

16. T. Østbye et al., "The Effect of the Home Environment on Physical Activity and Dietary Intake in Preschool Children," *International Journal of Obesity* 37, no. 10 (May 20, 2013): 1314–21, https://doi .org/10.1038/ijo.2013.76.

17. Jody Brumage, "The Public Health Cigarette Smoking Act of 1970," Robert C. Byrd Center for Congressional History and Education, July 25, 2017, https://www.byrdcenter.org/blog/ the-public-health-cigarette-smoking-act-of-1970.

18. Federal Trade Commission – Reports, "A Review of Food Marketing to Children and Adolescents: Follow-Up Report," December 2012, https://www.ftc.gov/sites/default/files/documents/reports/review-food-marketing-children-and-adolescents-follow -report/121221foodmarketingreport.pdf.

19. Center for Science in the Public Interest, "Food Marketing to Kids," last modified October 12, 2022, https://www.cspinet.org/advocacy/nutrition/food-marketing-kids.

20. Rebecca G. Boswell and Hedy Kober, "Food Cue Reactivity and Craving Predict Eating and Weight Gain: A Meta-Analytic Review," *Obesity Reviews* 17, no. 2 (February 2016): 159–77, https://doi.org/10.1111/obr.12354.

21. Jennifer R. Harris, John A. Bargh, and Kelly D. Brownell, "Priming Effects of Television Food Advertising on Eating Behavior," *Health Psychology* 28, no. 4 (January 1, 2009): 404–13, https://doi.org/10.1037/a0014399.

22. Sonia J. Miller et al., "Association between Television Viewing and Poor Diet Quality in Young Children," *Pediatric Obesity* 3, no. 3 (January 1, 2008): 168–76, https://doi.org/10.1080/17477160 801915935.

23. Eliza Barclay, "Scientists Are Building a Case for How Food Ads Make Us Overeat," NPR, January 29, 2016, https://www.npr.org/sections/thesalt/2016/01/29/462838153/food-ads-make-us-eat -more-and-should-be-regulated.

24. BBB National Programs, "Children's Food & Beverage Advertising Initiative," accessed December 4, 2023, https://bbbprograms.org/programs/all-programs/cfbai.

25. Melissa L. Jensen et al., "Food Industry Self-regulation: Changes in Nutrition of Foods and Drinks That May Be Advertised to Children," UConn Rudd Center for Food Policy & Health, April 2022, https://www.cacfp.org/assets/pdf/FACTS2022+Rudd +Report+Food+Marketing/.

26. Punam Ohri-Vachaspati et al., "Evidence That Changes in Community Food Environments Lead to Changes in Children's Weight: Results from a Longitudinal Prospective Cohort Study," *Journal of the Academy of Nutrition and Dietetics* 121, no. 3 (March 1, 2021): 419-34.e9, https://doi.org/10.1016/j.jand.2020.10.016.

27. Elisa Pineda et al., "The Retail Food Environment and Its Association with Body Mass Index in Mexico," *International Journal of Obesity* 45, no. 6 (February 17, 2021): 1215–28, https://doi.org/10.1038/s41366-021-00760-2.

28. Terri Box, "Farmers' Markets Prices Are Actually Cheaper than Buying Produce at the Grocery Store," WBIW.com, August 18, 2022, https://www.wbiw.com/2022/08/18/farmers-markets-prices-are-actually-cheaper-than-buying-produce-at-the-grocery-store.

29. School Nutrition Association, "School Meal Statistics," accessed December 4, 2023, https://schoolnutrition.org/about-school-meals/school-meal-statistics/.

30. Pourya Valizadeh and Barry M. Popkin, "The New School Food Standards and Nutrition of School Children: Direct and Indirect Effect Analysis," *Economics and Human Biology* 39 (December 1, 2020): 100918, https://doi.org/10.1016/j.ehb.2020.100918.

31. US Department of Agriculture Economic Research Service – Topics, "Definitions of Food Security," last modified October 25, 2023, https://www.ers.usda.gov/topics/food-nutrition-assistance/food-security-in-the-u-s/definitions-of-food-security/.

32. Rachel Bleiweiss-Sande et al., "Associations between Food Group Intake, Cognition, and Academic Achievement in Elementary Schoolchildren," *Nutrients* 11, no. 11 (November 9, 2019): 2722, https://doi.org/10.3390/nu11112722.

33. Cameron English, "Changing Our 'Food Environment' Doesn't Slash Obesity," American Council on Science and Health, April 25, 2022, https://www.acsh.org/news/2022/04/25/changing-our-food-environment-doesnt-slash-obesity-16266.

34. Ana I. Pereira and Andreia Oliveira, "Dietary Interventions to Prevent Childhood Obesity: A Literature Review," *Nutrients* 13, no. 10 (September 28, 2021): 3447, https://doi.org/10.3390/nu13103447.

35. Food and Agriculture Organization of the United Nations, "The State of Food Security and Nutrition in the World 2021: Transforming food systems for food security, improved nutrition and afforadable healthy diets for all," United Nations International Children's Emergency Fund, https://www.unicef.org/dominican republic/media/5196/file/The%20State%20of%20Food%20Security %20and%20Nutrition%20in%20the%20World%202021.pdf.

CHAPTER 9

1. National Institutes of Health – News Releases, "NIH Awards $170 Million for Precision Nutrition Study," January 20, 2022, https://www.nih.gov/news-events/news-releases/nih-awards-170-million-precision-nutrition-study.

2. Centers for Disease Control and Prevention, "Health and Economic Costs of Chronic Diseases," accessed October 29, 2023, https://www.cdc.gov/chronicdisease/about/costs/index.htm.

3. Bradley C. Johnston et al., "Unprocessed Red Meat and Processed Meat Consumption: Dietary Guideline Recommendations From the Nutritional Recommendations (NutriRECS) Consortium," *Annals of Internal Medicine* 171, no. 10 (October 1, 2019): 756, https://doi.org/10.7326/m19-1621.

4. Keren Papier et al., "Meat Consumption and Risk of Ischemic Heart Disease: A Systematic Review and Meta-Analysis," *Critical Reviews in Food Science and Nutrition* 63, no. 3 (July 20, 2021): 426–37, https://doi.org/10.1080/10408398.2021.1949575.

5. National Institutes of Health, "Estimates of Funding for Various Research, Condition, and Disease Categories (RCDC)," RePORT: Research Portfolio Online Reporting Tools, March 31, 2023, https://report.nih.gov/funding/categorical-spending.

6. NIH National Institute of Allergy and Infectious Diseases, "Big Grants SOP," September 14, 2022, https://www.niaid.nih.gov/research/big-grants-sop.

7. National Institutes of Health Office of Nutrition Research, "2020–2030 Strategic Plan for NIH Nutrition Research," July 23, 2023, https://dpcpsi.nih.gov/onr/strategic-plan.

8. Duff Wilson and Janet Roberts, "Special Report: How Washington Went Soft on Childhood Obesity," Reuters, April 27, 2012, https://www.reuters.com/article/us-usa-foodlobby/special-report-how-washington-went-soft-on-childhood-obesity-idUSBRE83Q0ED20120427.

9. "Regulations.Gov," n.d., https://www.regulations.gov/document/FNS-2020-0038-2936.

10. Duff Wilson and Janet Roberts, "Special Report."

11. Christopher Doering, "Where the Dollars Go: Lobbying a Big Business for Large Food and Beverage CPGs," Food Dive, December 6, 2021, https://www.fooddive.com/news/where-the-dollars-go-lobbying-a-big-business-for-large-food-and-beverage-c/607982/.

12. n.a., "Public Agrees on Obesity's Impact, Not Government's Role," Pew Research Center, November 12, 2013, https://www.pewresearch.org/politics/2013/11/12/public-agrees-on-obesitys-impact-not-governments-role/.

13. LA Times Archives, "Weighing a Soda Tax," Food, *Los Angeles Times*, September 26, 2009, https://www.latimes.com/archives/la-xpm-2009-sep-26-ed-soda26-story.html.

14. American Beverage Association – Education Resources (blog), "Beverage Taxes Just Don't Work!," February 21, 2020, https://www.americanbeverage.org/education-resources/blog/post/beverage-taxes-just-don-t-work/.

15. Michael M. Grynbaum, "New York's Ban on Big Sodas Is Rejected by Final Court," *New York Times*, June 26, 2014, https://www.nytimes.com/2014/06/27/nyregion/city-loses-final-appeal-on-limiting-sales-of-large-sodas.html.

16. Center for Science in the Public Interest, "Big Soda vs. Public Health (2016 Edition)," last modified September 1, 2016, https://www.cspinet.org/resource/big-soda-vs-public-health-1.

17. Yichen Zhong et al., "Sugar-Sweetened and Diet Beverage Consumption in Philadelphia One Year After the Beverage Tax," *International Journal of Environmental Research and Public Health*, 17, no. 4 (February 19, 2020): 1336, https://doi.org/10.3390/ijerph17041336.

18. Claudia Lee, "How Does Lobbying Impact Our Food and Agricultural Policies?," FoodUnfolded, last modified July 20, 2023, https://www.foodunfolded.com/article/how-does-lobbying-impact-our-food-and-agricultural-policies.

19. "Bills Lobbied by Center for Science in Public Interest, 2020," OpenSecrets, accessed October 29, 2023, https://www.opensecrets.org/federal-lobbying/clients/bills?cycle=2020&id=D000048461.

20. "Center for Science in Public Interest Profile: Summary," OpenSecrets, accessed October 29, 2023, https://www.opensecrets.org/orgs/center-for-science-in-public-interest/summary?id=D000048461.

21. Scott Bixby, "One of Amy Klobuchar's Biggest Backers Is 'the Worst Company in the World,'" *Daily Beast*, February 13, 2020, https://www.thedailybeast.com/one-of-amy-klobuchars-biggest-backers-is-the-worst-company-in-the-world.

22. "Food & Beverage Lobbying Profile: Lobbyists," OpenSecrets, accessed October 29, 2023, https://www.opensecrets.org/federal-lobbying/industries/lobbyists?cycle=2021&id=N01.

23. The Center for Consumer Freedom, "About Us," accessed October 29, 2023, https://consumerfreedom.com/about/.

24. US Department of Agriculture Food and Nutrition Service, "Proposed Updates to the School Nutrition Standards," accessed October 29, 2023, https://www.fns.usda.gov/cn/proposed-updates-school-nutrition-standards.

25. School Nutrition Association – News, "SNA Comments on USDA's Proposed Nutrition Standards," March 28, 2023, https://school nutrition.org/sna-news/sna-comments-on-usdas-proposed -nutrition-standards/.

26. US Department of Agriculture Food and Nutrition Service – News Item, "USDA Helps Schools Build Back Better, Issues Transitional Nutrition Standards for Coming School Years," February 4, 2022, https://www.fns.usda.gov/news-item/usda-0037.22.

27. Ron Nixon, "School Lunch Proposals Set Off a Dispute," *New York Times*, November 2, 2011, https://www.nytimes.com/2011/11/02/us/school-lunch-proposals-set-off-a-dispute.html.

28. Ron Nixon, "Congress Blocks New Rules on School Lunches," *New York Times*, November 16, 2011, https://www.nytimes.com/2011/11/16/us/politics/congress-blocks-new-rules-on-school-lunches.html.

29. Samantha Graff, Dale Kunkel, and Seth E. Mermin, "Government Can Regulate Food Advertising To Children Because Cognitive Research Shows That It Is Inherently Misleading," *Health Affairs* 31, no. 2 (February 1, 2012): 392–98, https://doi.org/10.1377/hlthaff.2011.0609.

30. "Focus on Food: Understanding Labeling and the First Amendment," National Agricultural Law Center, accessed December 2, 2022, https://nationalaglawcenter.org/focus-on -food-understanding-labeling-and-the-first-amendment/.

31. American Psychological Association – Reports, "Report of the APA Task Force on Advertising and Children," February 20, 2004, https://www.apa.org/pubs/reports/advertising-children.

32. Federal Trade Commission, "Press Release: Interagency Working Group Seeks Input on Proposed Voluntary Principles for Marketing Food to Children," July 29, 2022, https://www.ftc.gov/news-events/news/press-releases/2011/04/interagency-working-group-seeks-input-proposed-voluntary-principles-marketing-food-children.

33. Lyndsey Layton, "Industries Lobby against Voluntary Nutrition Guidelines for Food Marketed to Kids," *Washington Post*, July 9, 2011, https://www.washingtonpost.com/politics/industries-lobby-against-voluntary-nutrition-guidelines-for-food-marketed-to-kids/2011/07/08/gIQAZSZu5H_story.html.

34. "Lawmakers Attack Plan to Limit Food Ads to Kids," Reuters, October 14, 2011, https://www.reuters.com/article/us-advertising-children/lawmakers-attack-plan-to-limit-food-ads-to-kids-idUSTRE79D44G20111014.

35. "Sen. Dick Durbin: Campaign Finance Summary," OpenSecrets, accessed October 29, 2023, https://www.opensecrets.org/members-of-congress/dick-durbin/summary?cid=N00004981.

36. Michele Simon, "More Empty Recommendations on Junk Food Marketing to Children," Center for Food Safety, May 10, 2012, https://www.centerforfoodsafety.org/issues/308/food-safety/blog/1130/more-empty-recommendations-on-junk-food-marketing-to-children.

37. United States Environmental Protection Agency, "Summary of the Toxic Substances Control Act," last modified September 29, 2023, https://www.epa.gov/laws-regulations/summary-toxic-substances-control-act.

38. David Ewing Duncan, "Chemicals Within Us," *National Geographic*, May 3, 2021, https://www.nationalgeographic.com/science/article/chemicals-within-us.

39. Zhanyun Wang et al., "We Need a Global Science-Policy Body on Chemicals and Waste," *Science* 371, no. 6531 (February 19, 2021): 774–76, https://doi.org/10.1126/science.abe9090.

40. Environmental Protection Agency Office of Inspector General, "National Toxicology Program," Department of Health and Human Services, accessed October 29, 2023, https://archive.epa.gov/oig/catalog/web/html/167.html.

41. Sharon Lerner, "Toxic 'Reform' Law Will Gut State Rules on Dangerous Chemicals," The Intercept, April 29, 2019, https://theintercept.com/2016/01/11/toxic-reform-law-would-gut-state-rules-on-dangerous-chemicals/.

42. "H.R.2576 - Frank R. Lautenberg Chemical Safety for the 21st Century Act," Congress.Gov, accessed June 28, 2023, https://www.congress.gov/bill/114th-congress/house-bill/2576/text/.

43. Rebecca Trager, "US Chemical Industry Responsible for 25% of the Country's GDP," Chemistry World, July 27, 2022, https://www.chemistryworld.com/news/us-chemical-industry-responsible-for-25-of-the-countrys-gdp/4016016.article.

44. Sharon Lerner, "Toxic 'Reform' Law Will Gut State Rules."

45. Eric Lipton, "Tom Udall's Unlikely Alliance With the Chemical Industry," New York Times, March 7, 2015, https://www.nytimes.com/2015/03/07/us/tom-udalls-unlikely-alliance-with-the-chemical-industry.html.

46. "Chemical & Related Manufacturing Lobbying Profile," OpenSecrets, accessed October 29, 2023, https://www.opensecrets.org/federal-lobbying/industries/summary?cycle=2022&id=N13.

47. Tom Perkins, "How US Chemical Industry Lobbying and Cash Defeated Regulation in Trump Era," Guardian, April 26, 2021, https://www.theguardian.com/environment/2021/apr/26/us-chemical-companies-lobbying-donation-defeated-regulation.

48. "Chemical & Related Manufacturing: Top Contributors to Federal Candidates, Parties, and Outside Groups," OpenSecrets, accessed October 29, 2023, https://www.opensecrets.org/industries/contrib.php?cycle=2020&ind=n13.

49. United States Environmental Protection Agency, "Press Release: Biden-Harris Administration Proposes First-Ever National Standard to Protect Communities from PFAS in Drinking Water," March 14, 2023, https://www.epa.gov/newsreleases/biden-harris -administration-proposes-first-ever-national-standard-protect -communities.

50. Marion Nestle, "The Ironic Politics of Obesity," *Science* 299, no. 5608 (February 7, 2003): 781, https://doi.org/10.1126/science .299.5608.781.

CHAPTER 10

1. Joseph S. Nelson, "Mindful Eating: The Art of Presence While You Eat," *Diabetes Spectrum* 30, no. 3 (August 1, 2017): 171–74, https:// doi.org/10.2337/ds17-0015.

2. Yann Cornil, "Mind over Stomach: A Review of the Cognitive Drivers of Food Satiation," *Journal of the Association for Consumer Research* 2, no. 4 (October 1, 2017): 419–29, https://doi .org/10.1086/693111.

3. Joyce H. Lee et al., "United States Dietary Trends Since 1800: Lack of Association Between Saturated Fatty Acid Consumption and Non-Communicable Diseases," *Frontiers in Nutrition* 8 (January 13, 2022), https://doi.org/10.3389/fnut.2021.748847.

4. "Fast Food Market Size, Share, Trends & Growth, 2021–2028," Fortune Business Insights, accessed October 29, 2023, https://www .fortunebusinessinsights.com/fast-food-market-106482.

5. Kevin D. Hall and Scott Kahan, "Maintenance of Lost Weight and Long-Term Management of Obesity," *Medical Clinics of North America* 102, no. 1 (January 1, 2018): 183–97, https://doi.org/ 10.1016/j.mcna.2017.08.012.

6. James M. Anderson et al., "Long-Term Weight-Loss Maintenance: A Meta-Analysis of US Studies," *The American Journal of Clinical Nutrition* 74, no. 5 (November 1, 2001): 579–84, https://doi .org/10.1093/ajcn/74.5.579.

7. Evan M. Forman and Meghan L. Butryn, "A New Look at the Science of Weight Control: How Acceptance and Commitment Strategies Can Address the Challenge of Self-Regulation," *Appetite* 84 (January 1, 2015): 171–80, https://doi.org/10.1016/j.appet .2014.10.004.

8. Jane E. Brody, "Counting Calories? Your Weight-Loss Plan May Be Outdated," *New York Times*, February 7, 2013, https://www.nytimes .com/2011/07/19/health/19brody.html.

9. Michelle R. vanDellen, Jennifer Isherwood, and Julie E. Delose, "How Do People Define Moderation?," *Appetite* 101 (June 1, 2016): 156–62, https://doi.org/10.1016/j.appet.2016.03.010.

10. Isabel Cristina De Macedo et al., "The Influence of Palatable Diets in Reward System Activation: A Mini Review," *Advances in Pharmacological Sciences* 2016 (January 1, 2016): 1–7, https://doi .org/10.1155/2016/7238679.

11. Eran Magen et al., "Behavioral and Neural Correlates of Increased Self-Control in the Absence of Increased Willpower," *Proceedings of the National Academy of Sciences* 111, no. 27 (June 23, 2014): 9786–91, https://doi.org/10.1073/pnas.1408991111.

12. Roy F. Baumeister et al., "Ego Depletion: Is the Active Self a Limited Resource?" *Journal of Personality and Social Psychology* 74, no. 5 (January 1, 1998): 1252–65, https://doi.org/10.1037/0022 -3514.74.5.1252.

13. Hans Villarica, "The Chocolate-and-Radish Experiment That Birthed the Modern Conception of Willpower," *Atlantic*, April 9, 2012, https://www.theatlantic.com/health/archive/2012/04/the -chocolate-and-radish-experiment-that-birthed-the-modern -conception-of-willpower/255544/.

14. B. R. Beck, "Neuropeptide-Y in Normal Eating and in Genetic and Dietary-Induced Obesity," *Philosophical Transactions of the Royal Society* B 361, no. 1471 (June 19, 2006): 1159–85, https://doi.org/10.1098/rstb.2006.1855.

15. Kelley Strohacker et al., "Adaptations of Leptin, Ghrelin or Insulin during Weight Loss as Predictors of Weight Regain: A Review of Current Literature," *International Journal of Obesity* 38, no. 3 (June 26, 2013): 388–96, https://doi.org/10.1038/ijo.2013.118.

16. Gary W. Miller, "Appetite Regulation: Hormones, Peptides, and Neurotransmitters and Their Role in Obesity," *American Journal of Lifestyle Medicine* 13, no. 6 (June 23, 2017): 586–601, https://doi.org/10.1177/1559827617716376.

17. Angel E. Navidad, "Marshmallow Test Experiment and Delayed Gratification," Simply Psychology, May 1, 2023, https://www.simplypsychology.org/marshmallow-test.html.

18. Dan Ariely, *Predictably Irrational: The Hidden Forces That Shape Our Decisions*, revised and expanded ed. (New York: HarperCollins, 2010).

19. Alice S. Ammerman, Terry Hartman, and Molly DeMarco, "Behavioral Economics and the Supplemental Nutrition Assistance Program," *American Journal of Preventive Medicine* 52, no. 2 (February 1, 2017): S145–50, https://doi.org/10.1016/j.amepre.2016.08.017.

SECTION III

1. Radhika Gupta et al., "Endocrine Disruption and Obesity: A Current Review on Environmental Obesogens," *Current Research in Green and Sustainable Chemistry* 3 (June 1, 2020): 100009, https://doi.org/10.1016/j.crgsc.2020.06.002.

2. G. Frigerio, Chiara Ferrari, and Silvia Fustinoni, "Prenatal and Childhood Exposure to Per-/Polyfluoroalkyl Substances (PFASs) and Its Associations With Childhood Overweight and/or Obesity: A Systematic Review With Meta-analyses," *Environmental Health*, 22, no. 1 (August 14, 2023): https://doi.org/10.1186/s12940-023-01006-6.

3. Beate Leppert et al., "Maternal Paraben Exposure Triggers Childhood Overweight Development," *Nature Communications* 11, no. 1 (February 11, 2020), https://doi.org/10.1038/s41467-019 -14202-1.

4. Max Knoblauch, "Americans Feel Guilty about Almost a Third of the Food They Eat," *New York Post*, March 13, 2019, https:// nypost.com/2019/03/13/americans-feel-guilty-about-almost -a-third-of-the-food-they-eat/.

5. American Heart Association, "Yo-Yo Dieting Dangerous Even If You're Not Overweight," EurekAlert!, November 15, 2016, https:// www.eurekalert.org/news-releases/607702.

6. The Rochester Center for Behavioral Medicine (blog), "Nutrition Related Concerns for Women over Age 50," accessed December 4, 2023, https://www.rcbm.net/behavioral-medicine/blog-detail/ nutrition-related-concerns-for-women-over-age-50.

7. Janet Chrzan and Kima Cargill, *Anxious Eaters: Why We Fall for Fad Diets* (New York: Columbia University Press, 2022).

8. Rochelle Embling et al., "Effect of Food Variety on Intake of a Meal: A Systematic Review and Meta-Analysis," *The American Journal of Clinical Nutrition* 113, no. 3 (March 1, 2021): 716–41, https://doi.org/10.1093/ajcn/nqaa352.

9. Heather D. Whitehead et al., "Fluorinated Compounds in North American Cosmetics," *Environmental Science and Technology Letters* 8, no. 7 (June 15, 2021): 538–44, https://doi.org/10.1021/acs .estlett.1c00240.

10. Leppert et al., "Maternal Paraben Exposure."

11. Stephen Gullo, *The Thin Commandments Diet: The Ten No-Fail Strategies for Permanent Weight Loss* (New York: Random House Large Print Publishing, 2005), 29.

12. National Center for Complementary and Integrative Health, "Chelation for Coronary Heart Disease: What You Need To Know," accessed October 29, 2023, https://www.nccih.nih.gov/health/ chelation-for-coronary-heart-disease-what-you-need-to-know.

13. Nadia Barbo et al., "Locally Caught Freshwater Fish Across the United States Are Likely a Significant Source of Exposure to PFOS and Other Perfluorinated Compounds," *Environmental Research*, no. 220 (March 1, 2023): 115165, https://doi.org/10.1016/j.envres.2022.115165.

14. Rianne D. Stowell et al., "Noradrenergic Signaling in the Wakeful State Inhibits Microglial Surveillance and Synaptic Plasticity in the Mouse Visual Cortex," *Nature Neuroscience* 22, no. 11 (October 21, 2019): 1782–92, https://doi.org/10.1038/s41593-019-0514-0.

15. Steven C. Hayes et al., "Acceptance and Commitment Therapy: Model, Processes and Outcomes," *Behaviour Research and Therapy* 44, no. 1 (January 1, 2006): 1–25, https://doi.org/10.1016/j.brat.2005.06.006.

16. Daniel A. Assaz et al., "A Process-Based Analysis of Cognitive Defusion in Acceptance and Commitment Therapy," *Behavior Therapy* 54, no. 6 (November 2023): 1020–1035, https://doi.org/10.1016/j.beth.2022.06.003.

Index

About the Authors

As a leading player on the front lines against obesity, **STEWART LONKY, MD,** has devoted years to uncovering the effects of excess weight on human health. For nearly four decades, he has been a pioneering doctor with a thriving clinical, academic, and laboratory career. He writes and frequently speaks on the growing obesity and overweight epidemic and boasts impressive accomplishments. Visit drlonky.com to explore articles, blog posts, and insights related to obesity, weight management, and overall health.

Dr. Lonky is currently the medical director and founder of West Coast Cardiopulmonary, Inc., and heads a successful medical practice bearing his name. After earning his medical degree from Downstate Medical Center and completing an internship at Brooklyn's Kings County Hospital, Dr. Lonky was selected by Barnes Hospital (St. Louis) as a junior assistant resident before becoming a senior resident at the UC San Diego Medical Center, now UC San Diego Health. Dr. Lonky followed up with a National

Institutes of Health fellowship in pulmonary disease and biochemistry. Dr. Lonky regularly performs medical-legal evaluations, which are exams used to determine the cause, extent, and medical treatment of injuries where liability is in question. Additionally, Dr. Lonky holds an MBA from Pepperdine University. Dr. Lonky serves on the board of directors of the NutraPharma Corporation, and also the Histologics Corporation.

Dr. Lonky was among the first doctors to highlight the link between environmental pollutants and human health, and was the first doctor to publish peer-reviewed research on the efficacy of using an activated form of natural zeolite to help with the excretion of toxic metals from the human body. He also co-authored the book *Invisible Killers: The Truth About Environmental Genocide*.

He has been instrumental in raising the medical and lay communities' awareness of the connection between oxygen deprivation and right heart failure, a seldom-discussed topic in all the hype surrounding cardiovascular disease. Dr. Lonky's research, particularly the connection between oxygen deprivation and obesity, has opened the door to new possibilities for reducing weight-related morbidity and mortality.

Dr. Lonky is a diplomate of the American Boards of Internal Medicine, Pulmonary, and Critical Care Medicine and a member of the American College of Chest Physicians and the California Lung Association. In addition, he holds memberships in the American Thoracic Society and the American Federation for Clinical Research. He is a fellow of the American College of Physicians.

Dr. Lonky lives with his wife, Marilyn, in Los Angeles and Santa Barbara. They have two daughters and four grandchildren.

CHRIS TALLEY is a nutritional scientist specializing in the unique requirements of ultra-elite athletic performance. He has almost three decades of experience in the related fields of nutritional science and exercise physiology.

His career began in aerospace physiology, where he studied the effects of microgravity environmental conditions on human metabolic processes. He soon discovered that many of the nutritional interventions that helped preserve muscle mass and neurological function in space also increased muscle mass and sharpened nervous system performance on Earth. Mr. Talley parlayed his discovery into the world of peak athletic performance, which led to the founding of Precision Food Works, Inc. PFW uses a synergistic combination of blood/urinalysis and software to create a comprehensive, state-of-the-art dietary regimen. The software utilizes proprietary algorithms to generate personalized recipes that contain the precise quantity of protein, carbohydrate, and fat required to achieve each client's goals quickly and safely.

Past and current PFW clients include:

- Multiple Major League Baseball MVPs, four MLB Cy Young Award–winning pitchers, and more than thirty MLB All-Stars

- Several NBA MVPs and dozens of NBA All-Stars

- Two NFL MVPs

- Dozens of Professional Bowlers Association members

- Multiple Heisman Trophy winners

- Two world champion figure skaters

- Over twenty gold medal–winning Olympians

- Dozens of record-holding, world-class athletes

- Hundreds of actors, models, media personalities, and corporate executives

Mr. Talley is a frequent and featured speaker at nutritional seminars, and some of the world's most respected sports medicine physicians routinely seek his expertise. In addition, Mr. Talley was formerly Red Bull's high-performance nutrition counsel, ensuring that all company-sponsored, world-class athletes have the best dietary programs and advice possible. Mr. Talley has spoken at multiple Department of Defense symposiums focusing on using artificial intelligence software to find associations between lifestyle, diet, and hormone levels. Most recently, he was the keynote speaker at the 2023 Sports Cardiovascular and Nutrition (SCAN) symposium on artificial intelligence and dietetics.

Mr. Talley resides in Los Angeles.